AF882718

Diabetes Blood Sugar Record
and
Blood Pressure Log

This Book Belongs to:

Name_________________________________

Phone Number__________________________

Physician______________________________Phone____________________________

Physician______________________________Phone____________________________

Specialist______________________________Phone____________________________

Specialist______________________________Phone____________________________

Pharmacy_____________________________Phone_____________________________

Copyright © 2023 Himari Publishing. By Carol Bacon

All rights reserved. No part of this book may be reproduced in any form without written permission from the author or publisher, except as permitted by U.S. copyright law.

Table of Contents

Weekly Diabetes Blood Sugar Record

Target A1C: _______ My Current A1C: _______ Target Blood Sugar Before Meals: ______

Target Blood Sugar After Meals: _____ Physical Activity Goal: ____________________

Week of: ______________		Blood Sugar Level **Before**	Medication/ Insulin Dose	Blood Sugar Level **2 Hrs. After**	Physical Activity	Comments: Medication/Insulin taken How do you feel?
MONDAY					☐ Yes ☐ No	
MEAL	Time:					
☐ Breakfast						
☐ Lunch						
☐ Dinner						
☐ Snack						
		Blood Sugar Level **Before**	Medication/ Insulin Dose	Blood Sugar Level **2 Hrs. After**	Physical Activity	Comments: Medication/Insulin taken How do you feel?
TUESDAY					☐ Yes ☐ No	
MEAL	Time:					
☐ Breakfast						
☐ Lunch						
☐ Dinner						
☐ Snack						
		Blood Sugar Level **Before**	Medication/ Insulin Dose	Blood Sugar Level **2 Hrs. After**	Physical Activity	Comments: Medication/Insulin taken How do you feel?
WEDNESDAY					☐ Yes ☐ No	
MEAL	Time:					
☐ Breakfast						
☐ Lunch						
☐ Dinner						
☐ Snack						

Look for trends in your Diabetes Control. Take this record with you to your doctor visits.

		Blood Sugar Level **Before**	Medication/ Insulin Dose	Blood Sugar Level **2 Hrs. After**	Physical Activity	Comments: Medication/Insulin taken How do you feel?
THURSDAY					☐ Yes ☐ No	
MEAL	Time:					
☐ Breakfast						
☐ Lunch						
☐ Dinner						
☐ Snack						

		Blood Sugar Level **Before**	Medication/ Insulin Dose	Blood Sugar Level **2 Hrs. After**	Physical Activity	Comments: Medication/Insulin taken How do you feel?
FRIDAY					☐ Yes ☐ No	
MEAL	Time:					
☐ Breakfast						
☐ Lunch						
☐ Dinner						
☐ Snack						

		Blood Sugar Level **Before**	Medication/ Insulin Dose	Blood Sugar Level **2 Hrs. After**	Physical Activity	Comments: Medication/Insulin taken How do you feel?
SATURDAY					☐ Yes ☐ No	
MEAL	Time:					
☐ Breakfast						
☐ Lunch						
☐ Dinner						
☐ Snack						

		Blood Sugar Level **Before**	Medication/ Insulin Dose	Blood Sugar Level **2 Hrs. After**	Physical Activity	Comments: Medication/Insulin taken How do you feel?
SUNDAY					☐ Yes ☐ No	
MEAL	Time:					
☐ Breakfast						
☐ Lunch						
☐ Dinner						
☐ Snack						

Weekly Diabetes Blood Sugar Record

Target A1C: ______ My Current A1C: ______ Target Blood Sugar Before Meals: ______

Target Blood Sugar After Meals: _____ Physical Activity Goal: ____________________

Week of: ______________		Blood Sugar Level **Before**	Medication/ Insulin Dose	Blood Sugar Level **2 Hrs. After**	Physical Activity	Comments: Medication/Insulin taken How do you feel?
MONDAY					☐ Yes ☐ No	
MEAL	Time:					
☐ Breakfast						
☐ Lunch						
☐ Dinner						
☐ Snack						
		Blood Sugar Level **Before**	Medication/ Insulin Dose	Blood Sugar Level **2 Hrs. After**	Physical Activity	Comments: Medication/Insulin taken How do you feel?
TUESDAY					☐ Yes ☐ No	
MEAL	Time:					
☐ Breakfast						
☐ Lunch						
☐ Dinner						
☐ Snack						
		Blood Sugar Level **Before**	Medication/ Insulin Dose	Blood Sugar Level **2 Hrs. After**	Physical Activity	Comments: Medication/Insulin taken How do you feel?
WEDNESDAY					☐ Yes ☐ No	
MEAL	Time:					
☐ Breakfast						
☐ Lunch						
☐ Dinner						
☐ Snack						

	Blood Sugar Level **Before**	Medication/ Insulin Dose	Blood Sugar Level **2 Hrs. After**	Physical Activity	Comments: Medication/Insulin taken How do you feel?
THURSDAY				☐ Yes ☐ No	
MEAL Time:					
☐ Breakfast					
☐ Lunch					
☐ Dinner					
☐ Snack					

	Blood Sugar Level **Before**	Medication/ Insulin Dose	Blood Sugar Level **2 Hrs. After**	Physical Activity	Comments: Medication/Insulin taken How do you feel?
FRIDAY				☐ Yes ☐ No	
MEAL Time:					
☐ Breakfast					
☐ Lunch					
☐ Dinner					
☐ Snack					

	Blood Sugar Level **Before**	Medication/ Insulin Dose	Blood Sugar Level **2 Hrs. After**	Physical Activity	Comments: Medication/Insulin taken How do you feel?
SATURDAY				☐ Yes ☐ No	
MEAL Time:					
☐ Breakfast					
☐ Lunch					
☐ Dinner					
☐ Snack					

	Blood Sugar Level **Before**	Medication/ Insulin Dose	Blood Sugar Level **2 Hrs. After**	Physical Activity	Comments: Medication/Insulin taken How do you feel?
SUNDAY				☐ Yes ☐ No	
MEAL Time:					
☐ Breakfast					
☐ Lunch					
☐ Dinner					
☐ Snack					

Weekly Diabetes Blood Sugar Record

Target A1C: ______ My Current A1C: ______ Target Blood Sugar Before Meals: ______

Target Blood Sugar After Meals: _____ Physical Activity Goal: ____________________

Week of: ______________		Blood Sugar Level **Before**	Medication/ Insulin Dose	Blood Sugar Level **2 Hrs. After**	Physical Activity	Comments: Medication/Insulin taken How do you feel?
MONDAY					☐ Yes ☐ No	
MEAL	Time:					
☐ Breakfast						
☐ Lunch						
☐ Dinner						
☐ Snack						
		Blood Sugar Level **Before**	Medication/ Insulin Dose	Blood Sugar Level **2 Hrs. After**	Physical Activity	Comments: Medication/Insulin taken How do you feel?
TUESDAY					☐ Yes ☐ No	
MEAL	Time:					
☐ Breakfast						
☐ Lunch						
☐ Dinner						
☐ Snack						
		Blood Sugar Level **Before**	Medication/ Insulin Dose	Blood Sugar Level **2 Hrs. After**	Physical Activity	Comments: Medication/Insulin taken How do you feel?
WEDNESDAY					☐ Yes ☐ No	
MEAL	Time:					
☐ Breakfast						
☐ Lunch						
☐ Dinner						
☐ Snack						

		Blood Sugar Level **Before**	Medication/ Insulin Dose	Blood Sugar Level **2 Hrs. After**	Physical Activity	Comments: Medication/Insulin taken How do you feel?
THURSDAY					☐ Yes ☐ No	
MEAL	Time:					
☐ Breakfast						
☐ Lunch						
☐ Dinner						
☐ Snack						

		Blood Sugar Level **Before**	Medication/ Insulin Dose	Blood Sugar Level **2 Hrs. After**	Physical Activity	Comments: Medication/Insulin taken How do you feel?
FRIDAY					☐ Yes ☐ No	
MEAL	Time:					
☐ Breakfast						
☐ Lunch						
☐ Dinner						
☐ Snack						

		Blood Sugar Level **Before**	Medication/ Insulin Dose	Blood Sugar Level **2 Hrs. After**	Physical Activity	Comments: Medication/Insulin taken How do you feel?
SATURDAY					☐ Yes ☐ No	
MEAL	Time:					
☐ Breakfast						
☐ Lunch						
☐ Dinner						
☐ Snack						

		Blood Sugar Level **Before**	Medication/ Insulin Dose	Blood Sugar Level **2 Hrs. After**	Physical Activity	Comments: Medication/Insulin taken How do you feel?
SUNDAY					☐ Yes ☐ No	
MEAL	Time:					
☐ Breakfast						
☐ Lunch						
☐ Dinner						
☐ Snack						

Weekly Diabetes Blood Sugar Record

Target A1C: ______ My Current A1C: ______ Target Blood Sugar Before Meals: _____

Target Blood Sugar After Meals: _____ Physical Activity Goal: ____________________

Week of: ______________		Blood Sugar Level **Before**	Medication/ Insulin Dose	Blood Sugar Level **2 Hrs. After**	Physical Activity	Comments: Medication/Insulin taken How do you feel?
MONDAY					☐ Yes ☐ No	
MEAL	Time:					
☐ Breakfast						
☐ Lunch						
☐ Dinner						
☐ Snack						
		Blood Sugar Level **Before**	Medication/ Insulin Dose	Blood Sugar Level **2 Hrs. After**	Physical Activity	Comments: Medication/Insulin taken How do you feel?
TUESDAY					☐ Yes ☐ No	
MEAL	Time:					
☐ Breakfast						
☐ Lunch						
☐ Dinner						
☐ Snack						
		Blood Sugar Level **Before**	Medication/ Insulin Dose	Blood Sugar Level **2 Hrs. After**	Physical Activity	Comments: Medication/Insulin taken How do you feel?
WEDNESDAY					☐ Yes ☐ No	
MEAL	Time:					
☐ Breakfast						
☐ Lunch						
☐ Dinner						
☐ Snack						

		Blood Sugar Level **Before**	Medication/ Insulin Dose	Blood Sugar Level **2 Hrs. After**	Physical Activity	Comments: Medication/Insulin taken How do you feel?
THURSDAY					☐ Yes ☐ No	
MEAL	Time:					
☐ Breakfast						
☐ Lunch						
☐ Dinner						
☐ Snack						

		Blood Sugar Level **Before**	Medication/ Insulin Dose	Blood Sugar Level **2 Hrs. After**	Physical Activity	Comments: Medication/Insulin taken How do you feel?
FRIDAY					☐ Yes ☐ No	
MEAL	Time:					
☐ Breakfast						
☐ Lunch						
☐ Dinner						
☐ Snack						

		Blood Sugar Level **Before**	Medication/ Insulin Dose	Blood Sugar Level **2 Hrs. After**	Physical Activity	Comments: Medication/Insulin taken How do you feel?
SATURDAY					☐ Yes ☐ No	
MEAL	Time:					
☐ Breakfast						
☐ Lunch						
☐ Dinner						
☐ Snack						

		Blood Sugar Level **Before**	Medication/ Insulin Dose	Blood Sugar Level **2 Hrs. After**	Physical Activity	Comments: Medication/Insulin taken How do you feel?
SUNDAY					☐ Yes ☐ No	
MEAL	Time:					
☐ Breakfast						
☐ Lunch						
☐ Dinner						
☐ Snack						

Weekly Diabetes Blood Sugar Record

Target A1C: ______ My Current A1C: ______ Target Blood Sugar Before Meals: ______

Target Blood Sugar After Meals: _____ Physical Activity Goal: ____________________

Week of: ______________		Blood Sugar Level **Before**	Medication/ Insulin Dose	Blood Sugar Level **2 Hrs. After**	Physical Activity	Comments: Medication/Insulin taken How do you feel?
MONDAY					☐ Yes ☐ No	
MEAL	Time:					
☐ Breakfast						
☐ Lunch						
☐ Dinner						
☐ Snack						

		Blood Sugar Level **Before**	Medication/ Insulin Dose	Blood Sugar Level **2 Hrs. After**	Physical Activity	Comments: Medication/Insulin taken How do you feel?
TUESDAY					☐ Yes ☐ No	
MEAL	Time:					
☐ Breakfast						
☐ Lunch						
☐ Dinner						
☐ Snack						

		Blood Sugar Level **Before**	Medication/ Insulin Dose	Blood Sugar Level **2 Hrs. After**	Physical Activity	Comments: Medication/Insulin taken How do you feel?
WEDNESDAY					☐ Yes ☐ No	
MEAL	Time:					
☐ Breakfast						
☐ Lunch						
☐ Dinner						
☐ Snack						

		Blood Sugar Level **Before**	Medication/ Insulin Dose	Blood Sugar Level **2 Hrs. After**	Physical Activity	Comments: Medication/Insulin taken How do you feel?
THURSDAY					☐ Yes ☐ No	
MEAL	Time:					
☐ Breakfast						
☐ Lunch						
☐ Dinner						
☐ Snack						

		Blood Sugar Level **Before**	Medication/ Insulin Dose	Blood Sugar Level **2 Hrs. After**	Physical Activity	Comments: Medication/Insulin taken How do you feel?
FRIDAY					☐ Yes ☐ No	
MEAL	Time:					
☐ Breakfast						
☐ Lunch						
☐ Dinner						
☐ Snack						

		Blood Sugar Level **Before**	Medication/ Insulin Dose	Blood Sugar Level **2 Hrs. After**	Physical Activity	Comments: Medication/Insulin taken How do you feel?
SATURDAY					☐ Yes ☐ No	
MEAL	Time:					
☐ Breakfast						
☐ Lunch						
☐ Dinner						
☐ Snack						

		Blood Sugar Level **Before**	Medication/ Insulin Dose	Blood Sugar Level **2 Hrs. After**	Physical Activity	Comments: Medication/Insulin taken How do you feel?
SUNDAY					☐ Yes ☐ No	
MEAL	Time:					
☐ Breakfast						
☐ Lunch						
☐ Dinner						
☐ Snack						

Weekly Diabetes Blood Sugar Record

Target A1C: ______ My Current A1C: ______ Target Blood Sugar Before Meals: ______

Target Blood Sugar After Meals: _____ Physical Activity Goal: ____________________

Week of: ______________		Blood Sugar Level **Before**	Medication/ Insulin Dose	Blood Sugar Level **2 Hrs. After**	Physical Activity	Comments: Medication/Insulin taken How do you feel?
MONDAY					☐ Yes ☐ No	
MEAL	Time:					
☐ Breakfast						
☐ Lunch						
☐ Dinner						
☐ Snack						
		Blood Sugar Level **Before**	Medication/ Insulin Dose	Blood Sugar Level **2 Hrs. After**	Physical Activity	Comments: Medication/Insulin taken How do you feel?
TUESDAY					☐ Yes ☐ No	
MEAL	Time:					
☐ Breakfast						
☐ Lunch						
☐ Dinner						
☐ Snack						
		Blood Sugar Level **Before**	Medication/ Insulin Dose	Blood Sugar Level **2 Hrs. After**	Physical Activity	Comments: Medication/Insulin taken How do you feel?
WEDNESDAY					☐ Yes ☐ No	
MEAL	Time:					
☐ Breakfast						
☐ Lunch						
☐ Dinner						
☐ Snack						

		Blood Sugar Level **Before**	Medication/ Insulin Dose	Blood Sugar Level **2 Hrs. After**	Physical Activity	Comments: Medication/Insulin taken How do you feel?
THURSDAY					☐ Yes ☐ No	
MEAL	Time:					
☐ Breakfast						
☐ Lunch						
☐ Dinner						
☐ Snack						
		Blood Sugar Level **Before**	Medication/ Insulin Dose	Blood Sugar Level **2 Hrs. After**	Physical Activity	Comments: Medication/Insulin taken How do you feel?
FRIDAY					☐ Yes ☐ No	
MEAL	Time:					
☐ Breakfast						
☐ Lunch						
☐ Dinner						
☐ Snack						
		Blood Sugar Level **Before**	Medication/ Insulin Dose	Blood Sugar Level **2 Hrs. After**	Physical Activity	Comments: Medication/Insulin taken How do you feel?
SATURDAY					☐ Yes ☐ No	
MEAL	Time:					
☐ Breakfast						
☐ Lunch						
☐ Dinner						
☐ Snack						
		Blood Sugar Level **Before**	Medication/ Insulin Dose	Blood Sugar Level **2 Hrs. After**	Physical Activity	Comments: Medication/Insulin taken How do you feel?
SUNDAY					☐ Yes ☐ No	
MEAL	Time:					
☐ Breakfast						
☐ Lunch						
☐ Dinner						
☐ Snack						

Weekly Diabetes Blood Sugar Record

Target A1C: ______ My Current A1C: ______ Target Blood Sugar Before Meals: ______

Target Blood Sugar After Meals: _____ Physical Activity Goal: ____________________

Week of: ______________		Blood Sugar Level **Before**	Medication/ Insulin Dose	Blood Sugar Level **2 Hrs. After**	Physical Activity	Comments: Medication/Insulin taken How do you feel?
MONDAY					☐ Yes ☐ No	
MEAL	Time:					
☐ Breakfast						
☐ Lunch						
☐ Dinner						
☐ Snack						
		Blood Sugar Level **Before**	Medication/ Insulin Dose	Blood Sugar Level **2 Hrs. After**	Physical Activity	Comments: Medication/Insulin taken How do you feel?
TUESDAY					☐ Yes ☐ No	
MEAL	Time:					
☐ Breakfast						
☐ Lunch						
☐ Dinner						
☐ Snack						
		Blood Sugar Level **Before**	Medication/ Insulin Dose	Blood Sugar Level **2 Hrs. After**	Physical Activity	Comments: Medication/Insulin taken How do you feel?
WEDNESDAY					☐ Yes ☐ No	
MEAL	Time:					
☐ Breakfast						
☐ Lunch						
☐ Dinner						
☐ Snack						

	Blood Sugar Level **Before**	Medication/ Insulin Dose	Blood Sugar Level **2 Hrs. After**	Physical Activity	Comments: Medication/Insulin taken How do you feel?
THURSDAY				☐ Yes ☐ No	
MEAL Time:					
☐ Breakfast					
☐ Lunch					
☐ Dinner					
☐ Snack					
	Blood Sugar Level **Before**	Medication/ Insulin Dose	Blood Sugar Level **2 Hrs. After**	Physical Activity	Comments: Medication/Insulin taken How do you feel?
FRIDAY				☐ Yes ☐ No	
MEAL Time:					
☐ Breakfast					
☐ Lunch					
☐ Dinner					
☐ Snack					
	Blood Sugar Level **Before**	Medication/ Insulin Dose	Blood Sugar Level **2 Hrs. After**	Physical Activity	Comments: Medication/Insulin taken How do you feel?
SATURDAY				☐ Yes ☐ No	
MEAL Time:					
☐ Breakfast					
☐ Lunch					
☐ Dinner					
☐ Snack					
	Blood Sugar Level **Before**	Medication/ Insulin Dose	Blood Sugar Level **2 Hrs. After**	Physical Activity	Comments: Medication/Insulin taken How do you feel?
SUNDAY				☐ Yes ☐ No	
MEAL Time:					
☐ Breakfast					
☐ Lunch					
☐ Dinner					
☐ Snack					

Weekly Diabetes Blood Sugar Record

Target A1C: ______ My Current A1C: ______ Target Blood Sugar Before Meals: _____

Target Blood Sugar After Meals: _____ Physical Activity Goal: ____________________

Week of: ______________		Blood Sugar Level **Before**	Medication/ Insulin Dose	Blood Sugar Level **2 Hrs. After**	Physical Activity	Comments: Medication/Insulin taken How do you feel?
MONDAY					☐ Yes ☐ No	
MEAL	Time:					
☐ Breakfast						
☐ Lunch						
☐ Dinner						
☐ Snack						
		Blood Sugar Level **Before**	Medication/ Insulin Dose	Blood Sugar Level **2 Hrs. After**	Physical Activity	Comments: Medication/Insulin taken How do you feel?
TUESDAY					☐ Yes ☐ No	
MEAL	Time:					
☐ Breakfast						
☐ Lunch						
☐ Dinner						
☐ Snack						
		Blood Sugar Level **Before**	Medication/ Insulin Dose	Blood Sugar Level **2 Hrs. After**	Physical Activity	Comments: Medication/Insulin taken How do you feel?
WEDNESDAY					☐ Yes ☐ No	
MEAL	Time:					
☐ Breakfast						
☐ Lunch						
☐ Dinner						
☐ Snack						

	Blood Sugar Level **Before**	Medication/ Insulin Dose	Blood Sugar Level **2 Hrs. After**	Physical Activity	Comments: Medication/Insulin taken How do you feel?
THURSDAY				☐ Yes	
MEAL Time:				☐ No	
☐ Breakfast					
☐ Lunch					
☐ Dinner					
☐ Snack					

	Blood Sugar Level **Before**	Medication/ Insulin Dose	Blood Sugar Level **2 Hrs. After**	Physical Activity	Comments: Medication/Insulin taken How do you feel?
FRIDAY				☐ Yes	
MEAL Time:				☐ No	
☐ Breakfast					
☐ Lunch					
☐ Dinner					
☐ Snack					

	Blood Sugar Level **Before**	Medication/ Insulin Dose	Blood Sugar Level **2 Hrs. After**	Physical Activity	Comments: Medication/Insulin taken How do you feel?
SATURDAY				☐ Yes	
MEAL Time:				☐ No	
☐ Breakfast					
☐ Lunch					
☐ Dinner					
☐ Snack					

	Blood Sugar Level **Before**	Medication/ Insulin Dose	Blood Sugar Level **2 Hrs. After**	Physical Activity	Comments: Medication/Insulin taken How do you feel?
SUNDAY				☐ Yes	
MEAL Time:				☐ No	
☐ Breakfast					
☐ Lunch					
☐ Dinner					
☐ Snack					

Weekly Diabetes Blood Sugar Record

Target A1C: ______ My Current A1C: ______ Target Blood Sugar Before Meals: ______

Target Blood Sugar After Meals: _____ Physical Activity Goal: ____________________

Week of: ______________		Blood Sugar Level **Before**	Medication/ Insulin Dose	Blood Sugar Level **2 Hrs. After**	Physical Activity	Comments: Medication/Insulin taken How do you feel?
MONDAY					☐ Yes ☐ No	
MEAL	Time:					
☐ Breakfast						
☐ Lunch						
☐ Dinner						
☐ Snack						
		Blood Sugar Level **Before**	Medication/ Insulin Dose	Blood Sugar Level **2 Hrs. After**	Physical Activity	Comments: Medication/Insulin taken How do you feel?
TUESDAY					☐ Yes ☐ No	
MEAL	Time:					
☐ Breakfast						
☐ Lunch						
☐ Dinner						
☐ Snack						
		Blood Sugar Level **Before**	Medication/ Insulin Dose	Blood Sugar Level **2 Hrs. After**	Physical Activity	Comments: Medication/Insulin taken How do you feel?
WEDNESDAY					☐ Yes ☐ No	
MEAL	Time:					
☐ Breakfast						
☐ Lunch						
☐ Dinner						
☐ Snack						

		Blood Sugar Level **Before**	Medication/ Insulin Dose	Blood Sugar Level **2 Hrs. After**	Physical Activity	Comments: Medication/Insulin taken How do you feel?
THURSDAY					☐ Yes	
MEAL	Time:				☐ No	
☐ Breakfast						
☐ Lunch						
☐ Dinner						
☐ Snack						
		Blood Sugar Level **Before**	Medication/ Insulin Dose	Blood Sugar Level **2 Hrs. After**	Physical Activity	Comments: Medication/Insulin taken How do you feel?
FRIDAY					☐ Yes	
MEAL	Time:				☐ No	
☐ Breakfast						
☐ Lunch						
☐ Dinner						
☐ Snack						
		Blood Sugar Level **Before**	Medication/ Insulin Dose	Blood Sugar Level **2 Hrs. After**	Physical Activity	Comments: Medication/Insulin taken How do you feel?
SATURDAY					☐ Yes	
MEAL	Time:				☐ No	
☐ Breakfast						
☐ Lunch						
☐ Dinner						
☐ Snack						
		Blood Sugar Level **Before**	Medication/ Insulin Dose	Blood Sugar Level **2 Hrs. After**	Physical Activity	Comments: Medication/Insulin taken How do you feel?
SUNDAY					☐ Yes	
MEAL	Time:				☐ No	
☐ Breakfast						
☐ Lunch						
☐ Dinner						
☐ Snack						

Weekly Diabetes Blood Sugar Record

Target A1C: ______ My Current A1C: ______ Target Blood Sugar Before Meals: _____

Target Blood Sugar After Meals: _____ Physical Activity Goal: ____________________

Week of: ______________		Blood Sugar Level **Before**	Medication/ Insulin Dose	Blood Sugar Level **2 Hrs. After**	Physical Activity	Comments: Medication/Insulin taken How do you feel?
MONDAY					☐ Yes	
MEAL	Time:				☐ No	
☐ Breakfast						
☐ Lunch						
☐ Dinner						
☐ Snack						
		Blood Sugar Level **Before**	Medication/ Insulin Dose	Blood Sugar Level **2 Hrs. After**	Physical Activity	Comments: Medication/Insulin taken How do you feel?
TUESDAY					☐ Yes	
MEAL	Time:				☐ No	
☐ Breakfast						
☐ Lunch						
☐ Dinner						
☐ Snack						
		Blood Sugar Level **Before**	Medication/ Insulin Dose	Blood Sugar Level **2 Hrs. After**	Physical Activity	Comments: Medication/Insulin taken How do you feel?
WEDNESDAY					☐ Yes	
MEAL	Time:				☐ No	
☐ Breakfast						
☐ Lunch						
☐ Dinner						
☐ Snack						

		Blood Sugar Level **Before**	Medication/ Insulin Dose	Blood Sugar Level **2 Hrs. After**	Physical Activity	Comments: Medication/Insulin taken How do you feel?
THURSDAY					☐ Yes ☐ No	
MEAL	Time:					
☐ Breakfast						
☐ Lunch						
☐ Dinner						
☐ Snack						

		Blood Sugar Level **Before**	Medication/ Insulin Dose	Blood Sugar Level **2 Hrs. After**	Physical Activity	Comments: Medication/Insulin taken How do you feel?
FRIDAY					☐ Yes ☐ No	
MEAL	Time:					
☐ Breakfast						
☐ Lunch						
☐ Dinner						
☐ Snack						

		Blood Sugar Level **Before**	Medication/ Insulin Dose	Blood Sugar Level **2 Hrs. After**	Physical Activity	Comments: Medication/Insulin taken How do you feel?
SATURDAY					☐ Yes ☐ No	
MEAL	Time:					
☐ Breakfast						
☐ Lunch						
☐ Dinner						
☐ Snack						

		Blood Sugar Level **Before**	Medication/ Insulin Dose	Blood Sugar Level **2 Hrs. After**	Physical Activity	Comments: Medication/Insulin taken How do you feel?
SUNDAY					☐ Yes ☐ No	
MEAL	Time:					
☐ Breakfast						
☐ Lunch						
☐ Dinner						
☐ Snack						

Weekly Diabetes Blood Sugar Record

Target A1C: _______ My Current A1C: _______ Target Blood Sugar Before Meals: ______

Target Blood Sugar After Meals: _____ Physical Activity Goal: ____________________

Week of: ____________		Blood Sugar Level **Before**	Medication/ Insulin Dose	Blood Sugar Level **2 Hrs. After**	Physical Activity	Comments: Medication/Insulin taken How do you feel?
MONDAY					☐ Yes ☐ No	
MEAL	Time:					
☐ Breakfast						
☐ Lunch						
☐ Dinner						
☐ Snack						
		Blood Sugar Level **Before**	Medication/ Insulin Dose	Blood Sugar Level **2 Hrs. After**	Physical Activity	Comments: Medication/Insulin taken How do you feel?
TUESDAY					☐ Yes ☐ No	
MEAL	Time:					
☐ Breakfast						
☐ Lunch						
☐ Dinner						
☐ Snack						
		Blood Sugar Level **Before**	Medication/ Insulin Dose	Blood Sugar Level **2 Hrs. After**	Physical Activity	Comments: Medication/Insulin taken How do you feel?
WEDNESDAY					☐ Yes ☐ No	
MEAL	Time:					
☐ Breakfast						
☐ Lunch						
☐ Dinner						
☐ Snack						

		Blood Sugar Level **Before**	Medication/ Insulin Dose	Blood Sugar Level **2 Hrs. After**	Physical Activity	Comments: Medication/Insulin taken How do you feel?
THURSDAY					☐ Yes ☐ No	
MEAL	Time:					
☐ Breakfast						
☐ Lunch						
☐ Dinner						
☐ Snack						

		Blood Sugar Level **Before**	Medication/ Insulin Dose	Blood Sugar Level **2 Hrs. After**	Physical Activity	Comments: Medication/Insulin taken How do you feel?
FRIDAY					☐ Yes ☐ No	
MEAL	Time:					
☐ Breakfast						
☐ Lunch						
☐ Dinner						
☐ Snack						

		Blood Sugar Level **Before**	Medication/ Insulin Dose	Blood Sugar Level **2 Hrs. After**	Physical Activity	Comments: Medication/Insulin taken How do you feel?
SATURDAY					☐ Yes ☐ No	
MEAL	Time:					
☐ Breakfast						
☐ Lunch						
☐ Dinner						
☐ Snack						

		Blood Sugar Level **Before**	Medication/ Insulin Dose	Blood Sugar Level **2 Hrs. After**	Physical Activity	Comments: Medication/Insulin taken How do you feel?
SUNDAY					☐ Yes ☐ No	
MEAL	Time:					
☐ Breakfast						
☐ Lunch						
☐ Dinner						
☐ Snack						

Weekly Diabetes Blood Sugar Record

Target A1C: ______ My Current A1C: ______ Target Blood Sugar Before Meals: ______

Target Blood Sugar After Meals: _____ Physical Activity Goal: ____________________

Week of: ______________		Blood Sugar Level **Before**	Medication/ Insulin Dose	Blood Sugar Level **2 Hrs. After**	Physical Activity	Comments: Medication/Insulin taken How do you feel?
MONDAY					☐ Yes ☐ No	
MEAL	Time:					
☐ Breakfast						
☐ Lunch						
☐ Dinner						
☐ Snack						
		Blood Sugar Level **Before**	Medication/ Insulin Dose	Blood Sugar Level **2 Hrs. After**	Physical Activity	Comments: Medication/Insulin taken How do you feel?
TUESDAY					☐ Yes ☐ No	
MEAL	Time:					
☐ Breakfast						
☐ Lunch						
☐ Dinner						
☐ Snack						
		Blood Sugar Level **Before**	Medication/ Insulin Dose	Blood Sugar Level **2 Hrs. After**	Physical Activity	Comments: Medication/Insulin taken How do you feel?
WEDNESDAY					☐ Yes ☐ No	
MEAL	Time:					
☐ Breakfast						
☐ Lunch						
☐ Dinner						
☐ Snack						

		Blood Sugar Level **Before**	Medication/ Insulin Dose	Blood Sugar Level **2 Hrs. After**	Physical Activity	Comments: Medication/Insulin taken How do you feel?
THURSDAY					☐ Yes ☐ No	
MEAL	Time:					
☐ Breakfast						
☐ Lunch						
☐ Dinner						
☐ Snack						
		Blood Sugar Level **Before**	Medication/ Insulin Dose	Blood Sugar Level **2 Hrs. After**	Physical Activity	Comments: Medication/Insulin taken How do you feel?
FRIDAY					☐ Yes ☐ No	
MEAL	Time:					
☐ Breakfast						
☐ Lunch						
☐ Dinner						
☐ Snack						
		Blood Sugar Level **Before**	Medication/ Insulin Dose	Blood Sugar Level **2 Hrs. After**	Physical Activity	Comments: Medication/Insulin taken How do you feel?
SATURDAY					☐ Yes ☐ No	
MEAL	Time:					
☐ Breakfast						
☐ Lunch						
☐ Dinner						
☐ Snack						
		Blood Sugar Level **Before**	Medication/ Insulin Dose	Blood Sugar Level **2 Hrs. After**	Physical Activity	Comments: Medication/Insulin taken How do you feel?
SUNDAY					☐ Yes ☐ No	
MEAL	Time:					
☐ Breakfast						
☐ Lunch						
☐ Dinner						
☐ Snack						

Weekly Diabetes Blood Sugar Record

Target A1C: ______ My Current A1C: ______ Target Blood Sugar Before Meals: ______

Target Blood Sugar After Meals: _____ Physical Activity Goal: ____________________

Week of: ______________		Blood Sugar Level **Before**	Medication/ Insulin Dose	Blood Sugar Level **2 Hrs. After**	Physical Activity	Comments: Medication/Insulin taken How do you feel?
MONDAY					☐ Yes ☐ No	
MEAL	Time:					
☐ Breakfast						
☐ Lunch						
☐ Dinner						
☐ Snack						
		Blood Sugar Level **Before**	Medication/ Insulin Dose	Blood Sugar Level **2 Hrs. After**	Physical Activity	Comments: Medication/Insulin taken How do you feel?
TUESDAY					☐ Yes ☐ No	
MEAL	Time:					
☐ Breakfast						
☐ Lunch						
☐ Dinner						
☐ Snack						
		Blood Sugar Level **Before**	Medication/ Insulin Dose	Blood Sugar Level **2 Hrs. After**	Physical Activity	Comments: Medication/Insulin taken How do you feel?
WEDNESDAY					☐ Yes ☐ No	
MEAL	Time:					
☐ Breakfast						
☐ Lunch						
☐ Dinner						
☐ Snack						

	Blood Sugar Level **Before**	Medication/ Insulin Dose	Blood Sugar Level **2 Hrs. After**	Physical Activity	Comments: Medication/Insulin taken How do you feel?
THURSDAY				☐ Yes ☐ No	
MEAL Time:					
☐ Breakfast					
☐ Lunch					
☐ Dinner					
☐ Snack					
	Blood Sugar Level **Before**	Medication/ Insulin Dose	Blood Sugar Level **2 Hrs. After**	Physical Activity	Comments: Medication/Insulin taken How do you feel?
FRIDAY				☐ Yes ☐ No	
MEAL Time:					
☐ Breakfast					
☐ Lunch					
☐ Dinner					
☐ Snack					
	Blood Sugar Level **Before**	Medication/ Insulin Dose	Blood Sugar Level **2 Hrs. After**	Physical Activity	Comments: Medication/Insulin taken How do you feel?
SATURDAY				☐ Yes ☐ No	
MEAL Time:					
☐ Breakfast					
☐ Lunch					
☐ Dinner					
☐ Snack					
	Blood Sugar Level **Before**	Medication/ Insulin Dose	Blood Sugar Level **2 Hrs. After**	Physical Activity	Comments: Medication/Insulin taken How do you feel?
SUNDAY				☐ Yes ☐ No	
MEAL Time:					
☐ Breakfast					
☐ Lunch					
☐ Dinner					
☐ Snack					

Weekly Diabetes Blood Sugar Record

Target A1C: ______ My Current A1C: ______ Target Blood Sugar Before Meals: _____

Target Blood Sugar After Meals: _____ Physical Activity Goal: ____________________

Week of: ______________		Blood Sugar Level **Before**	Medication/ Insulin Dose	Blood Sugar Level **2 Hrs. After**	Physical Activity	Comments: Medication/Insulin taken How do you feel?
MONDAY					☐ Yes ☐ No	
MEAL	Time:					
☐ Breakfast						
☐ Lunch						
☐ Dinner						
☐ Snack						
		Blood Sugar Level **Before**	Medication/ Insulin Dose	Blood Sugar Level **2 Hrs. After**	Physical Activity	Comments: Medication/Insulin taken How do you feel?
TUESDAY					☐ Yes ☐ No	
MEAL	Time:					
☐ Breakfast						
☐ Lunch						
☐ Dinner						
☐ Snack						
		Blood Sugar Level **Before**	Medication/ Insulin Dose	Blood Sugar Level **2 Hrs. After**	Physical Activity	Comments: Medication/Insulin taken How do you feel?
WEDNESDAY					☐ Yes ☐ No	
MEAL	Time:					
☐ Breakfast						
☐ Lunch						
☐ Dinner						
☐ Snack						

	Blood Sugar Level **Before**	Medication/ Insulin Dose	Blood Sugar Level **2 Hrs. After**	Physical Activity	Comments: Medication/Insulin taken How do you feel?
THURSDAY				☐ Yes ☐ No	
MEAL Time:					
☐ Breakfast					
☐ Lunch					
☐ Dinner					
☐ Snack					
	Blood Sugar Level **Before**	Medication/ Insulin Dose	Blood Sugar Level **2 Hrs. After**	Physical Activity	Comments: Medication/Insulin taken How do you feel?
FRIDAY				☐ Yes ☐ No	
MEAL Time:					
☐ Breakfast					
☐ Lunch					
☐ Dinner					
☐ Snack					
	Blood Sugar Level **Before**	Medication/ Insulin Dose	Blood Sugar Level **2 Hrs. After**	Physical Activity	Comments: Medication/Insulin taken How do you feel?
SATURDAY				☐ Yes ☐ No	
MEAL Time:					
☐ Breakfast					
☐ Lunch					
☐ Dinner					
☐ Snack					
	Blood Sugar Level **Before**	Medication/ Insulin Dose	Blood Sugar Level **2 Hrs. After**	Physical Activity	Comments: Medication/Insulin taken How do you feel?
SUNDAY				☐ Yes ☐ No	
MEAL Time:					
☐ Breakfast					
☐ Lunch					
☐ Dinner					
☐ Snack					

Weekly Diabetes Blood Sugar Record

Target A1C: ______ My Current A1C: ______ Target Blood Sugar Before Meals: ______

Target Blood Sugar After Meals: _____ Physical Activity Goal: ____________________

Week of: ______________		Blood Sugar Level **Before**	Medication/ Insulin Dose	Blood Sugar Level **2 Hrs. After**	Physical Activity	Comments: Medication/Insulin taken How do you feel?
MONDAY					☐ Yes ☐ No	
MEAL	Time:					
☐ Breakfast						
☐ Lunch						
☐ Dinner						
☐ Snack						
		Blood Sugar Level **Before**	Medication/ Insulin Dose	Blood Sugar Level **2 Hrs. After**	Physical Activity	Comments: Medication/Insulin taken How do you feel?
TUESDAY					☐ Yes ☐ No	
MEAL	Time:					
☐ Breakfast						
☐ Lunch						
☐ Dinner						
☐ Snack						
		Blood Sugar Level **Before**	Medication/ Insulin Dose	Blood Sugar Level **2 Hrs. After**	Physical Activity	Comments: Medication/Insulin taken How do you feel?
WEDNESDAY					☐ Yes ☐ No	
MEAL	Time:					
☐ Breakfast						
☐ Lunch						
☐ Dinner						
☐ Snack						

	Blood Sugar Level **Before**	Medication/ Insulin Dose	Blood Sugar Level **2 Hrs. After**	Physical Activity	Comments: Medication/Insulin taken How do you feel?
THURSDAY				☐ Yes ☐ No	
MEAL Time:					
☐ Breakfast					
☐ Lunch					
☐ Dinner					
☐ Snack					

	Blood Sugar Level **Before**	Medication/ Insulin Dose	Blood Sugar Level **2 Hrs. After**	Physical Activity	Comments: Medication/Insulin taken How do you feel?
FRIDAY				☐ Yes ☐ No	
MEAL Time:					
☐ Breakfast					
☐ Lunch					
☐ Dinner					
☐ Snack					

	Blood Sugar Level **Before**	Medication/ Insulin Dose	Blood Sugar Level **2 Hrs. After**	Physical Activity	Comments: Medication/Insulin taken How do you feel?
SATURDAY				☐ Yes ☐ No	
MEAL Time:					
☐ Breakfast					
☐ Lunch					
☐ Dinner					
☐ Snack					

	Blood Sugar Level **Before**	Medication/ Insulin Dose	Blood Sugar Level **2 Hrs. After**	Physical Activity	Comments: Medication/Insulin taken How do you feel?
SUNDAY				☐ Yes ☐ No	
MEAL Time:					
☐ Breakfast					
☐ Lunch					
☐ Dinner					
☐ Snack					

Weekly Diabetes Blood Sugar Record

Target A1C: ______ My Current A1C: ______ Target Blood Sugar Before Meals: ______

Target Blood Sugar After Meals: _____ Physical Activity Goal: ____________________

Week of: ______________		Blood Sugar Level **Before**	Medication/ Insulin Dose	Blood Sugar Level **2 Hrs. After**	Physical Activity	Comments: Medication/Insulin taken How do you feel?
MONDAY					☐ Yes	
MEAL	Time:				☐ No	
☐ Breakfast						
☐ Lunch						
☐ Dinner						
☐ Snack						
		Blood Sugar Level **Before**	Medication/ Insulin Dose	Blood Sugar Level **2 Hrs. After**	Physical Activity	Comments: Medication/Insulin taken How do you feel?
TUESDAY					☐ Yes	
MEAL	Time:				☐ No	
☐ Breakfast						
☐ Lunch						
☐ Dinner						
☐ Snack						
		Blood Sugar Level **Before**	Medication/ Insulin Dose	Blood Sugar Level **2 Hrs. After**	Physical Activity	Comments: Medication/Insulin taken How do you feel?
WEDNESDAY					☐ Yes	
MEAL	Time:				☐ No	
☐ Breakfast						
☐ Lunch						
☐ Dinner						
☐ Snack						

		Blood Sugar Level **Before**	Medication/ Insulin Dose	Blood Sugar Level **2 Hrs. After**	Physical Activity	Comments: Medication/Insulin taken How do you feel?
THURSDAY					☐ Yes ☐ No	
MEAL	Time:					
☐ Breakfast						
☐ Lunch						
☐ Dinner						
☐ Snack						
		Blood Sugar Level **Before**	Medication/ Insulin Dose	Blood Sugar Level **2 Hrs. After**	Physical Activity	Comments: Medication/Insulin taken How do you feel?
FRIDAY					☐ Yes ☐ No	
MEAL	Time:					
☐ Breakfast						
☐ Lunch						
☐ Dinner						
☐ Snack						
		Blood Sugar Level **Before**	Medication/ Insulin Dose	Blood Sugar Level **2 Hrs. After**	Physical Activity	Comments: Medication/Insulin taken How do you feel?
SATURDAY					☐ Yes ☐ No	
MEAL	Time:					
☐ Breakfast						
☐ Lunch						
☐ Dinner						
☐ Snack						
		Blood Sugar Level **Before**	Medication/ Insulin Dose	Blood Sugar Level **2 Hrs. After**	Physical Activity	Comments: Medication/Insulin taken How do you feel?
SUNDAY					☐ Yes ☐ No	
MEAL	Time:					
☐ Breakfast						
☐ Lunch						
☐ Dinner						
☐ Snack						

Weekly Diabetes Blood Sugar Record

Target A1C: ______ My Current A1C: ______ Target Blood Sugar Before Meals: ______

Target Blood Sugar After Meals: _____ Physical Activity Goal: ____________________

Week of: ______________		Blood Sugar Level **Before**	Medication/ Insulin Dose	Blood Sugar Level **2 Hrs. After**	Physical Activity	Comments: Medication/Insulin taken How do you feel?
MONDAY					☐ Yes ☐ No	
MEAL	Time:					
☐ Breakfast						
☐ Lunch						
☐ Dinner						
☐ Snack						
		Blood Sugar Level **Before**	Medication/ Insulin Dose	Blood Sugar Level **2 Hrs. After**	Physical Activity	Comments: Medication/Insulin taken How do you feel?
TUESDAY					☐ Yes ☐ No	
MEAL	Time:					
☐ Breakfast						
☐ Lunch						
☐ Dinner						
☐ Snack						
		Blood Sugar Level **Before**	Medication/ Insulin Dose	Blood Sugar Level **2 Hrs. After**	Physical Activity	Comments: Medication/Insulin taken How do you feel?
WEDNESDAY					☐ Yes ☐ No	
MEAL	Time:					
☐ Breakfast						
☐ Lunch						
☐ Dinner						
☐ Snack						

	Blood Sugar Level **Before**	Medication/ Insulin Dose	Blood Sugar Level **2 Hrs. After**	Physical Activity	Comments: Medication/Insulin taken How do you feel?
THURSDAY				☐ Yes ☐ No	
MEAL Time:					
☐ Breakfast					
☐ Lunch					
☐ Dinner					
☐ Snack					

	Blood Sugar Level **Before**	Medication/ Insulin Dose	Blood Sugar Level **2 Hrs. After**	Physical Activity	Comments: Medication/Insulin taken How do you feel?
FRIDAY				☐ Yes ☐ No	
MEAL Time:					
☐ Breakfast					
☐ Lunch					
☐ Dinner					
☐ Snack					

	Blood Sugar Level **Before**	Medication/ Insulin Dose	Blood Sugar Level **2 Hrs. After**	Physical Activity	Comments: Medication/Insulin taken How do you feel?
SATURDAY				☐ Yes ☐ No	
MEAL Time:					
☐ Breakfast					
☐ Lunch					
☐ Dinner					
☐ Snack					

	Blood Sugar Level **Before**	Medication/ Insulin Dose	Blood Sugar Level **2 Hrs. After**	Physical Activity	Comments: Medication/Insulin taken How do you feel?
SUNDAY				☐ Yes ☐ No	
MEAL Time:					
☐ Breakfast					
☐ Lunch					
☐ Dinner					
☐ Snack					

Weekly Diabetes Blood Sugar Record

Target A1C: ______ My Current A1C: ______ Target Blood Sugar Before Meals: _____

Target Blood Sugar After Meals: _____ Physical Activity Goal: ____________________

Week of: ______________		Blood Sugar Level **Before**	Medication/ Insulin Dose	Blood Sugar Level **2 Hrs. After**	Physical Activity	Comments: Medication/Insulin taken How do you feel?
MONDAY					☐ Yes ☐ No	
MEAL	Time:					
☐ Breakfast						
☐ Lunch						
☐ Dinner						
☐ Snack						
		Blood Sugar Level **Before**	Medication/ Insulin Dose	Blood Sugar Level **2 Hrs. After**	Physical Activity	Comments: Medication/Insulin taken How do you feel?
TUESDAY					☐ Yes ☐ No	
MEAL	Time:					
☐ Breakfast						
☐ Lunch						
☐ Dinner						
☐ Snack						
		Blood Sugar Level **Before**	Medication/ Insulin Dose	Blood Sugar Level **2 Hrs. After**	Physical Activity	Comments: Medication/Insulin taken How do you feel?
WEDNESDAY					☐ Yes ☐ No	
MEAL	Time:					
☐ Breakfast						
☐ Lunch						
☐ Dinner						
☐ Snack						

		Blood Sugar Level **Before**	Medication/ Insulin Dose	Blood Sugar Level **2 Hrs. After**	Physical Activity	Comments: Medication/Insulin taken How do you feel?
THURSDAY					☐ Yes ☐ No	
MEAL	Time:					
☐ Breakfast						
☐ Lunch						
☐ Dinner						
☐ Snack						

		Blood Sugar Level **Before**	Medication/ Insulin Dose	Blood Sugar Level **2 Hrs. After**	Physical Activity	Comments: Medication/Insulin taken How do you feel?
FRIDAY					☐ Yes ☐ No	
MEAL	Time:					
☐ Breakfast						
☐ Lunch						
☐ Dinner						
☐ Snack						

		Blood Sugar Level **Before**	Medication/ Insulin Dose	Blood Sugar Level **2 Hrs. After**	Physical Activity	Comments: Medication/Insulin taken How do you feel?
SATURDAY					☐ Yes ☐ No	
MEAL	Time:					
☐ Breakfast						
☐ Lunch						
☐ Dinner						
☐ Snack						

		Blood Sugar Level **Before**	Medication/ Insulin Dose	Blood Sugar Level **2 Hrs. After**	Physical Activity	Comments: Medication/Insulin taken How do you feel?
SUNDAY					☐ Yes ☐ No	
MEAL	Time:					
☐ Breakfast						
☐ Lunch						
☐ Dinner						
☐ Snack						

Weekly Diabetes Blood Sugar Record

Target A1C: ______ My Current A1C: ______ Target Blood Sugar Before Meals: ______

Target Blood Sugar After Meals: _____ Physical Activity Goal: ____________________

Week of: ______________		Blood Sugar Level **Before**	Medication/ Insulin Dose	Blood Sugar Level **2 Hrs. After**	Physical Activity	Comments: Medication/Insulin taken How do you feel?
MONDAY					☐ Yes ☐ No	
MEAL	Time:					
☐ Breakfast						
☐ Lunch						
☐ Dinner						
☐ Snack						
		Blood Sugar Level **Before**	Medication/ Insulin Dose	Blood Sugar Level **2 Hrs. After**	Physical Activity	Comments: Medication/Insulin taken How do you feel?
TUESDAY					☐ Yes ☐ No	
MEAL	Time:					
☐ Breakfast						
☐ Lunch						
☐ Dinner						
☐ Snack						
		Blood Sugar Level **Before**	Medication/ Insulin Dose	Blood Sugar Level **2 Hrs. After**	Physical Activity	Comments: Medication/Insulin taken How do you feel?
WEDNESDAY					☐ Yes ☐ No	
MEAL	Time:					
☐ Breakfast						
☐ Lunch						
☐ Dinner						
☐ Snack						

	Blood Sugar Level **Before**	Medication/ Insulin Dose	Blood Sugar Level **2 Hrs. After**	Physical Activity	Comments: Medication/Insulin taken How do you feel?
THURSDAY				☐ Yes ☐ No	
MEAL Time:					
☐ Breakfast					
☐ Lunch					
☐ Dinner					
☐ Snack					

	Blood Sugar Level **Before**	Medication/ Insulin Dose	Blood Sugar Level **2 Hrs. After**	Physical Activity	Comments: Medication/Insulin taken How do you feel?
FRIDAY				☐ Yes ☐ No	
MEAL Time:					
☐ Breakfast					
☐ Lunch					
☐ Dinner					
☐ Snack					

	Blood Sugar Level **Before**	Medication/ Insulin Dose	Blood Sugar Level **2 Hrs. After**	Physical Activity	Comments: Medication/Insulin taken How do you feel?
SATURDAY				☐ Yes ☐ No	
MEAL Time:					
☐ Breakfast					
☐ Lunch					
☐ Dinner					
☐ Snack					

	Blood Sugar Level **Before**	Medication/ Insulin Dose	Blood Sugar Level **2 Hrs. After**	Physical Activity	Comments: Medication/Insulin taken How do you feel?
SUNDAY				☐ Yes ☐ No	
MEAL Time:					
☐ Breakfast					
☐ Lunch					
☐ Dinner					
☐ Snack					

Weekly Diabetes Blood Sugar Record

Target A1C: ______ My Current A1C: ______ Target Blood Sugar Before Meals: ______

Target Blood Sugar After Meals: _____ Physical Activity Goal: ____________________

Week of: ______________		Blood Sugar Level **Before**	Medication/ Insulin Dose	Blood Sugar Level **2 Hrs. After**	Physical Activity	Comments: Medication/Insulin taken How do you feel?
MONDAY					☐ Yes ☐ No	
MEAL	Time:					
☐ Breakfast						
☐ Lunch						
☐ Dinner						
☐ Snack						
		Blood Sugar Level **Before**	Medication/ Insulin Dose	Blood Sugar Level **2 Hrs. After**	Physical Activity	Comments: Medication/Insulin taken How do you feel?
TUESDAY					☐ Yes ☐ No	
MEAL	Time:					
☐ Breakfast						
☐ Lunch						
☐ Dinner						
☐ Snack						
		Blood Sugar Level **Before**	Medication/ Insulin Dose	Blood Sugar Level **2 Hrs. After**	Physical Activity	Comments: Medication/Insulin taken How do you feel?
WEDNESDAY					☐ Yes ☐ No	
MEAL	Time:					
☐ Breakfast						
☐ Lunch						
☐ Dinner						
☐ Snack						

	Blood Sugar Level **Before**	Medication/ Insulin Dose	Blood Sugar Level **2 Hrs. After**	Physical Activity	Comments: Medication/Insulin taken How do you feel?
THURSDAY				☐ Yes ☐ No	
MEAL Time:					
☐ Breakfast					
☐ Lunch					
☐ Dinner					
☐ Snack					

	Blood Sugar Level **Before**	Medication/ Insulin Dose	Blood Sugar Level **2 Hrs. After**	Physical Activity	Comments: Medication/Insulin taken How do you feel?
FRIDAY				☐ Yes ☐ No	
MEAL Time:					
☐ Breakfast					
☐ Lunch					
☐ Dinner					
☐ Snack					

	Blood Sugar Level **Before**	Medication/ Insulin Dose	Blood Sugar Level **2 Hrs. After**	Physical Activity	Comments: Medication/Insulin taken How do you feel?
SATURDAY				☐ Yes ☐ No	
MEAL Time:					
☐ Breakfast					
☐ Lunch					
☐ Dinner					
☐ Snack					

	Blood Sugar Level **Before**	Medication/ Insulin Dose	Blood Sugar Level **2 Hrs. After**	Physical Activity	Comments: Medication/Insulin taken How do you feel?
SUNDAY				☐ Yes ☐ No	
MEAL Time:					
☐ Breakfast					
☐ Lunch					
☐ Dinner					
☐ Snack					

Weekly Diabetes Blood Sugar Record

Target A1C: _______ My Current A1C: _______ Target Blood Sugar Before Meals: ______

Target Blood Sugar After Meals: _____ Physical Activity Goal: ______________________

Week of: ______________		Blood Sugar Level **Before**	Medication/ Insulin Dose	Blood Sugar Level **2 Hrs. After**	Physical Activity	Comments: Medication/Insulin taken How do you feel?
MONDAY					☐ Yes ☐ No	
MEAL	Time:					
☐ Breakfast						
☐ Lunch						
☐ Dinner						
☐ Snack						
		Blood Sugar Level **Before**	Medication/ Insulin Dose	Blood Sugar Level **2 Hrs. After**	Physical Activity	Comments: Medication/Insulin taken How do you feel?
TUESDAY					☐ Yes ☐ No	
MEAL	Time:					
☐ Breakfast						
☐ Lunch						
☐ Dinner						
☐ Snack						
		Blood Sugar Level **Before**	Medication/ Insulin Dose	Blood Sugar Level **2 Hrs. After**	Physical Activity	Comments: Medication/Insulin taken How do you feel?
WEDNESDAY					☐ Yes ☐ No	
MEAL	Time:					
☐ Breakfast						
☐ Lunch						
☐ Dinner						
☐ Snack						

		Blood Sugar Level **Before**	Medication/ Insulin Dose	Blood Sugar Level **2 Hrs. After**	Physical Activity	Comments: Medication/Insulin taken How do you feel?
THURSDAY					☐ Yes ☐ No	
MEAL	Time:					
☐ Breakfast						
☐ Lunch						
☐ Dinner						
☐ Snack						
		Blood Sugar Level **Before**	Medication/ Insulin Dose	Blood Sugar Level **2 Hrs. After**	Physical Activity	Comments: Medication/Insulin taken How do you feel?
FRIDAY					☐ Yes ☐ No	
MEAL	Time:					
☐ Breakfast						
☐ Lunch						
☐ Dinner						
☐ Snack						
		Blood Sugar Level **Before**	Medication/ Insulin Dose	Blood Sugar Level **2 Hrs. After**	Physical Activity	Comments: Medication/Insulin taken How do you feel?
SATURDAY					☐ Yes ☐ No	
MEAL	Time:					
☐ Breakfast						
☐ Lunch						
☐ Dinner						
☐ Snack						
		Blood Sugar Level **Before**	Medication/ Insulin Dose	Blood Sugar Level **2 Hrs. After**	Physical Activity	Comments: Medication/Insulin taken How do you feel?
SUNDAY					☐ Yes ☐ No	
MEAL	Time:					
☐ Breakfast						
☐ Lunch						
☐ Dinner						
☐ Snack						

Weekly Diabetes Blood Sugar Record

Target A1C: ______ My Current A1C: ______ Target Blood Sugar Before Meals: ______

Target Blood Sugar After Meals: _____ Physical Activity Goal: ____________________

Week of: ______________		Blood Sugar Level **Before**	Medication/ Insulin Dose	Blood Sugar Level **2 Hrs. After**	Physical Activity	Comments: Medication/Insulin taken How do you feel?
MONDAY					☐ Yes	
MEAL	Time:				☐ No	
☐ Breakfast						
☐ Lunch						
☐ Dinner						
☐ Snack						
		Blood Sugar Level **Before**	Medication/ Insulin Dose	Blood Sugar Level **2 Hrs. After**	Physical Activity	Comments: Medication/Insulin taken How do you feel?
TUESDAY					☐ Yes	
MEAL	Time:				☐ No	
☐ Breakfast						
☐ Lunch						
☐ Dinner						
☐ Snack						
		Blood Sugar Level **Before**	Medication/ Insulin Dose	Blood Sugar Level **2 Hrs. After**	Physical Activity	Comments: Medication/Insulin taken How do you feel?
WEDNESDAY					☐ Yes	
MEAL	Time:				☐ No	
☐ Breakfast						
☐ Lunch						
☐ Dinner						
☐ Snack						

		Blood Sugar Level **Before**	Medication/ Insulin Dose	Blood Sugar Level **2 Hrs. After**	Physical Activity	Comments: Medication/Insulin taken How do you feel?
THURSDAY					☐ Yes ☐ No	
MEAL	Time:					
☐ Breakfast						
☐ Lunch						
☐ Dinner						
☐ Snack						

		Blood Sugar Level **Before**	Medication/ Insulin Dose	Blood Sugar Level **2 Hrs. After**	Physical Activity	Comments: Medication/Insulin taken How do you feel?
FRIDAY					☐ Yes ☐ No	
MEAL	Time:					
☐ Breakfast						
☐ Lunch						
☐ Dinner						
☐ Snack						

		Blood Sugar Level **Before**	Medication/ Insulin Dose	Blood Sugar Level **2 Hrs. After**	Physical Activity	Comments: Medication/Insulin taken How do you feel?
SATURDAY					☐ Yes ☐ No	
MEAL	Time:					
☐ Breakfast						
☐ Lunch						
☐ Dinner						
☐ Snack						

		Blood Sugar Level **Before**	Medication/ Insulin Dose	Blood Sugar Level **2 Hrs. After**	Physical Activity	Comments: Medication/Insulin taken How do you feel?
SUNDAY					☐ Yes ☐ No	
MEAL	Time:					
☐ Breakfast						
☐ Lunch						
☐ Dinner						
☐ Snack						

Weekly Diabetes Blood Sugar Record

Target A1C: ______ My Current A1C: ______ Target Blood Sugar Before Meals: ______

Target Blood Sugar After Meals: _____ Physical Activity Goal: ____________________

Week of: ______________		Blood Sugar Level **Before**	Medication/ Insulin Dose	Blood Sugar Level **2 Hrs. After**	Physical Activity	Comments: Medication/Insulin taken How do you feel?
MONDAY					☐ Yes ☐ No	
MEAL	Time:					
☐ Breakfast						
☐ Lunch						
☐ Dinner						
☐ Snack						
		Blood Sugar Level **Before**	Medication/ Insulin Dose	Blood Sugar Level **2 Hrs. After**	Physical Activity	Comments: Medication/Insulin taken How do you feel?
TUESDAY					☐ Yes ☐ No	
MEAL	Time:					
☐ Breakfast						
☐ Lunch						
☐ Dinner						
☐ Snack						
		Blood Sugar Level **Before**	Medication/ Insulin Dose	Blood Sugar Level **2 Hrs. After**	Physical Activity	Comments: Medication/Insulin taken How do you feel?
WEDNESDAY					☐ Yes ☐ No	
MEAL	Time:					
☐ Breakfast						
☐ Lunch						
☐ Dinner						
☐ Snack						

		Blood Sugar Level **Before**	Medication/ Insulin Dose	Blood Sugar Level **2 Hrs. After**	Physical Activity	Comments: Medication/Insulin taken How do you feel?
THURSDAY					☐ Yes ☐ No	
MEAL	Time:					
☐ Breakfast						
☐ Lunch						
☐ Dinner						
☐ Snack						

		Blood Sugar Level **Before**	Medication/ Insulin Dose	Blood Sugar Level **2 Hrs. After**	Physical Activity	Comments: Medication/Insulin taken How do you feel?
FRIDAY					☐ Yes ☐ No	
MEAL	Time:					
☐ Breakfast						
☐ Lunch						
☐ Dinner						
☐ Snack						

		Blood Sugar Level **Before**	Medication/ Insulin Dose	Blood Sugar Level **2 Hrs. After**	Physical Activity	Comments: Medication/Insulin taken How do you feel?
SATURDAY					☐ Yes ☐ No	
MEAL	Time:					
☐ Breakfast						
☐ Lunch						
☐ Dinner						
☐ Snack						

		Blood Sugar Level **Before**	Medication/ Insulin Dose	Blood Sugar Level **2 Hrs. After**	Physical Activity	Comments: Medication/Insulin taken How do you feel?
SUNDAY					☐ Yes ☐ No	
MEAL	Time:					
☐ Breakfast						
☐ Lunch						
☐ Dinner						
☐ Snack						

Weekly Diabetes Blood Sugar Record

Target A1C: ______ My Current A1C: ______ Target Blood Sugar Before Meals: ______

Target Blood Sugar After Meals: _____ Physical Activity Goal: ____________________

Week of: ____________	Blood Sugar Level **Before**	Medication/ Insulin Dose	Blood Sugar Level **2 Hrs. After**	Physical Activity	Comments: Medication/Insulin taken How do you feel?
MONDAY				☐ Yes ☐ No	
MEAL Time:					
☐ Breakfast					
☐ Lunch					
☐ Dinner					
☐ Snack					
	Blood Sugar Level **Before**	Medication/ Insulin Dose	Blood Sugar Level **2 Hrs. After**	Physical Activity	Comments: Medication/Insulin taken How do you feel?
TUESDAY				☐ Yes ☐ No	
MEAL Time:					
☐ Breakfast					
☐ Lunch					
☐ Dinner					
☐ Snack					
	Blood Sugar Level **Before**	Medication/ Insulin Dose	Blood Sugar Level **2 Hrs. After**	Physical Activity	Comments: Medication/Insulin taken How do you feel?
WEDNESDAY				☐ Yes ☐ No	
MEAL Time:					
☐ Breakfast					
☐ Lunch					
☐ Dinner					
☐ Snack					

		Blood Sugar Level **Before**	Medication/ Insulin Dose	Blood Sugar Level **2 Hrs. After**	Physical Activity	Comments: Medication/Insulin taken How do you feel?
THURSDAY					☐ Yes ☐ No	
MEAL	Time:					
☐ Breakfast						
☐ Lunch						
☐ Dinner						
☐ Snack						
		Blood Sugar Level **Before**	Medication/ Insulin Dose	Blood Sugar Level **2 Hrs. After**	Physical Activity	Comments: Medication/Insulin taken How do you feel?
FRIDAY					☐ Yes ☐ No	
MEAL	Time:					
☐ Breakfast						
☐ Lunch						
☐ Dinner						
☐ Snack						
		Blood Sugar Level **Before**	Medication/ Insulin Dose	Blood Sugar Level **2 Hrs. After**	Physical Activity	Comments: Medication/Insulin taken How do you feel?
SATURDAY					☐ Yes ☐ No	
MEAL	Time:					
☐ Breakfast						
☐ Lunch						
☐ Dinner						
☐ Snack						
		Blood Sugar Level **Before**	Medication/ Insulin Dose	Blood Sugar Level **2 Hrs. After**	Physical Activity	Comments: Medication/Insulin taken How do you feel?
SUNDAY					☐ Yes ☐ No	
MEAL	Time:					
☐ Breakfast						
☐ Lunch						
☐ Dinner						
☐ Snack						

Weekly Diabetes Blood Sugar Record

Target A1C: ______ My Current A1C: ______ Target Blood Sugar Before Meals: ______

Target Blood Sugar After Meals: _____ Physical Activity Goal: ____________________

Week of: ____________		Blood Sugar Level **Before**	Medication/ Insulin Dose	Blood Sugar Level **2 Hrs. After**	Physical Activity	Comments: Medication/Insulin taken How do you feel?
MONDAY					☐ Yes	
MEAL	Time:				☐ No	
☐ Breakfast						
☐ Lunch						
☐ Dinner						
☐ Snack						
		Blood Sugar Level **Before**	Medication/ Insulin Dose	Blood Sugar Level **2 Hrs. After**	Physical Activity	Comments: Medication/Insulin taken How do you feel?
TUESDAY					☐ Yes	
MEAL	Time:				☐ No	
☐ Breakfast						
☐ Lunch						
☐ Dinner						
☐ Snack						
		Blood Sugar Level **Before**	Medication/ Insulin Dose	Blood Sugar Level **2 Hrs. After**	Physical Activity	Comments: Medication/Insulin taken How do you feel?
WEDNESDAY					☐ Yes	
MEAL	Time:				☐ No	
☐ Breakfast						
☐ Lunch						
☐ Dinner						
☐ Snack						

		Blood Sugar Level **Before**	Medication/ Insulin Dose	Blood Sugar Level **2 Hrs. After**	Physical Activity	Comments: Medication/Insulin taken How do you feel?
THURSDAY					☐ Yes ☐ No	
MEAL	Time:					
☐ Breakfast						
☐ Lunch						
☐ Dinner						
☐ Snack						
		Blood Sugar Level **Before**	Medication/ Insulin Dose	Blood Sugar Level **2 Hrs. After**	Physical Activity	Comments: Medication/Insulin taken How do you feel?
FRIDAY					☐ Yes ☐ No	
MEAL	Time:					
☐ Breakfast						
☐ Lunch						
☐ Dinner						
☐ Snack						
		Blood Sugar Level **Before**	Medication/ Insulin Dose	Blood Sugar Level **2 Hrs. After**	Physical Activity	Comments: Medication/Insulin taken How do you feel?
SATURDAY					☐ Yes ☐ No	
MEAL	Time:					
☐ Breakfast						
☐ Lunch						
☐ Dinner						
☐ Snack						
		Blood Sugar Level **Before**	Medication/ Insulin Dose	Blood Sugar Level **2 Hrs. After**	Physical Activity	Comments: Medication/Insulin taken How do you feel?
SUNDAY					☐ Yes ☐ No	
MEAL	Time:					
☐ Breakfast						
☐ Lunch						
☐ Dinner						
☐ Snack						

Weekly Diabetes Blood Sugar Record

Target A1C: ______ My Current A1C: ______ Target Blood Sugar Before Meals: ______

Target Blood Sugar After Meals: _____ Physical Activity Goal: ____________________

Week of: ______________		Blood Sugar Level **Before**	Medication/ Insulin Dose	Blood Sugar Level **2 Hrs. After**	Physical Activity	Comments: Medication/Insulin taken How do you feel?
MONDAY					☐ Yes ☐ No	
MEAL	Time:					
☐ Breakfast						
☐ Lunch						
☐ Dinner						
☐ Snack						

		Blood Sugar Level **Before**	Medication/ Insulin Dose	Blood Sugar Level **2 Hrs. After**	Physical Activity	Comments: Medication/Insulin taken How do you feel?
TUESDAY					☐ Yes ☐ No	
MEAL	Time:					
☐ Breakfast						
☐ Lunch						
☐ Dinner						
☐ Snack						

		Blood Sugar Level **Before**	Medication/ Insulin Dose	Blood Sugar Level **2 Hrs. After**	Physical Activity	Comments: Medication/Insulin taken How do you feel?
WEDNESDAY					☐ Yes ☐ No	
MEAL	Time:					
☐ Breakfast						
☐ Lunch						
☐ Dinner						
☐ Snack						

	Blood Sugar Level **Before**	Medication/ Insulin Dose	Blood Sugar Level **2 Hrs. After**	Physical Activity	Comments: Medication/Insulin taken How do you feel?
THURSDAY				☐ Yes ☐ No	
MEAL Time:					
☐ Breakfast					
☐ Lunch					
☐ Dinner					
☐ Snack					

	Blood Sugar Level **Before**	Medication/ Insulin Dose	Blood Sugar Level **2 Hrs. After**	Physical Activity	Comments: Medication/Insulin taken How do you feel?
FRIDAY				☐ Yes ☐ No	
MEAL Time:					
☐ Breakfast					
☐ Lunch					
☐ Dinner					
☐ Snack					

	Blood Sugar Level **Before**	Medication/ Insulin Dose	Blood Sugar Level **2 Hrs. After**	Physical Activity	Comments: Medication/Insulin taken How do you feel?
SATURDAY				☐ Yes ☐ No	
MEAL Time:					
☐ Breakfast					
☐ Lunch					
☐ Dinner					
☐ Snack					

	Blood Sugar Level **Before**	Medication/ Insulin Dose	Blood Sugar Level **2 Hrs. After**	Physical Activity	Comments: Medication/Insulin taken How do you feel?
SUNDAY				☐ Yes ☐ No	
MEAL Time:					
☐ Breakfast					
☐ Lunch					
☐ Dinner					
☐ Snack					

Weekly Diabetes Blood Sugar Record

Target A1C: ______ My Current A1C: ______ Target Blood Sugar Before Meals: ______

Target Blood Sugar After Meals: _____ Physical Activity Goal: ____________________

Week of: ______________		Blood Sugar Level **Before**	Medication/ Insulin Dose	Blood Sugar Level **2 Hrs. After**	Physical Activity	Comments: Medication/Insulin taken How do you feel?
MONDAY					☐ Yes ☐ No	
MEAL	Time:					
☐ Breakfast						
☐ Lunch						
☐ Dinner						
☐ Snack						
		Blood Sugar Level **Before**	Medication/ Insulin Dose	Blood Sugar Level **2 Hrs. After**	Physical Activity	Comments: Medication/Insulin taken How do you feel?
TUESDAY					☐ Yes ☐ No	
MEAL	Time:					
☐ Breakfast						
☐ Lunch						
☐ Dinner						
☐ Snack						
		Blood Sugar Level **Before**	Medication/ Insulin Dose	Blood Sugar Level **2 Hrs. After**	Physical Activity	Comments: Medication/Insulin taken How do you feel?
WEDNESDAY					☐ Yes ☐ No	
MEAL	Time:					
☐ Breakfast						
☐ Lunch						
☐ Dinner						
☐ Snack						

	Blood Sugar Level **Before**	Medication/ Insulin Dose	Blood Sugar Level **2 Hrs. After**	Physical Activity	Comments: Medication/Insulin taken How do you feel?
THURSDAY				☐ Yes ☐ No	
MEAL Time:					
☐ Breakfast					
☐ Lunch					
☐ Dinner					
☐ Snack					

	Blood Sugar Level **Before**	Medication/ Insulin Dose	Blood Sugar Level **2 Hrs. After**	Physical Activity	Comments: Medication/Insulin taken How do you feel?
FRIDAY				☐ Yes ☐ No	
MEAL Time:					
☐ Breakfast					
☐ Lunch					
☐ Dinner					
☐ Snack					

	Blood Sugar Level **Before**	Medication/ Insulin Dose	Blood Sugar Level **2 Hrs. After**	Physical Activity	Comments: Medication/Insulin taken How do you feel?
SATURDAY				☐ Yes ☐ No	
MEAL Time:					
☐ Breakfast					
☐ Lunch					
☐ Dinner					
☐ Snack					

	Blood Sugar Level **Before**	Medication/ Insulin Dose	Blood Sugar Level **2 Hrs. After**	Physical Activity	Comments: Medication/Insulin taken How do you feel?
SUNDAY				☐ Yes ☐ No	
MEAL Time:					
☐ Breakfast					
☐ Lunch					
☐ Dinner					
☐ Snack					

Weekly Diabetes Blood Sugar Record

Target A1C: ______ My Current A1C: ______ Target Blood Sugar Before Meals: _____

Target Blood Sugar After Meals: _____ Physical Activity Goal: ____________________

Week of: ______________		Blood Sugar Level **Before**	Medication/ Insulin Dose	Blood Sugar Level **2 Hrs. After**	Physical Activity	Comments: Medication/Insulin taken How do you feel?
MONDAY					☐ Yes ☐ No	
MEAL	Time:					
☐ Breakfast						
☐ Lunch						
☐ Dinner						
☐ Snack						
		Blood Sugar Level **Before**	Medication/ Insulin Dose	Blood Sugar Level **2 Hrs. After**	Physical Activity	Comments: Medication/Insulin taken How do you feel?
TUESDAY					☐ Yes ☐ No	
MEAL	Time:					
☐ Breakfast						
☐ Lunch						
☐ Dinner						
☐ Snack						
		Blood Sugar Level **Before**	Medication/ Insulin Dose	Blood Sugar Level **2 Hrs. After**	Physical Activity	Comments: Medication/Insulin taken How do you feel?
WEDNESDAY					☐ Yes ☐ No	
MEAL	Time:					
☐ Breakfast						
☐ Lunch						
☐ Dinner						
☐ Snack						

	Blood Sugar Level **Before**	Medication/ Insulin Dose	Blood Sugar Level **2 Hrs. After**	Physical Activity	Comments: Medication/Insulin taken How do you feel?
THURSDAY				☐ Yes ☐ No	
MEAL Time:					
☐ Breakfast					
☐ Lunch					
☐ Dinner					
☐ Snack					
	Blood Sugar Level **Before**	Medication/ Insulin Dose	Blood Sugar Level **2 Hrs. After**	Physical Activity	Comments: Medication/Insulin taken How do you feel?
FRIDAY				☐ Yes ☐ No	
MEAL Time:					
☐ Breakfast					
☐ Lunch					
☐ Dinner					
☐ Snack					
	Blood Sugar Level **Before**	Medication/ Insulin Dose	Blood Sugar Level **2 Hrs. After**	Physical Activity	Comments: Medication/Insulin taken How do you feel?
SATURDAY				☐ Yes ☐ No	
MEAL Time:					
☐ Breakfast					
☐ Lunch					
☐ Dinner					
☐ Snack					
	Blood Sugar Level **Before**	Medication/ Insulin Dose	Blood Sugar Level **2 Hrs. After**	Physical Activity	Comments: Medication/Insulin taken How do you feel?
SUNDAY				☐ Yes ☐ No	
MEAL Time:					
☐ Breakfast					
☐ Lunch					
☐ Dinner					
☐ Snack					

Weekly Diabetes Blood Sugar Record

Target A1C: ______ My Current A1C: ______ Target Blood Sugar Before Meals: ______

Target Blood Sugar After Meals: _____ Physical Activity Goal: ____________________

Week of: ______________		Blood Sugar Level **Before**	Medication/ Insulin Dose	Blood Sugar Level **2 Hrs. After**	Physical Activity	Comments: Medication/Insulin taken How do you feel?
MONDAY					☐ Yes ☐ No	
MEAL	Time:					
☐ Breakfast						
☐ Lunch						
☐ Dinner						
☐ Snack						
		Blood Sugar Level **Before**	Medication/ Insulin Dose	Blood Sugar Level **2 Hrs. After**	Physical Activity	Comments: Medication/Insulin taken How do you feel?
TUESDAY					☐ Yes ☐ No	
MEAL	Time:					
☐ Breakfast						
☐ Lunch						
☐ Dinner						
☐ Snack						
		Blood Sugar Level **Before**	Medication/ Insulin Dose	Blood Sugar Level **2 Hrs. After**	Physical Activity	Comments: Medication/Insulin taken How do you feel?
WEDNESDAY					☐ Yes ☐ No	
MEAL	Time:					
☐ Breakfast						
☐ Lunch						
☐ Dinner						
☐ Snack						

		Blood Sugar Level **Before**	Medication/ Insulin Dose	Blood Sugar Level **2 Hrs. After**	Physical Activity	Comments: Medication/Insulin taken How do you feel?
THURSDAY					☐ Yes ☐ No	
MEAL	Time:					
☐ Breakfast						
☐ Lunch						
☐ Dinner						
☐ Snack						

		Blood Sugar Level **Before**	Medication/ Insulin Dose	Blood Sugar Level **2 Hrs. After**	Physical Activity	Comments: Medication/Insulin taken How do you feel?
FRIDAY					☐ Yes ☐ No	
MEAL	Time:					
☐ Breakfast						
☐ Lunch						
☐ Dinner						
☐ Snack						

		Blood Sugar Level **Before**	Medication/ Insulin Dose	Blood Sugar Level **2 Hrs. After**	Physical Activity	Comments: Medication/Insulin taken How do you feel?
SATURDAY					☐ Yes ☐ No	
MEAL	Time:					
☐ Breakfast						
☐ Lunch						
☐ Dinner						
☐ Snack						

		Blood Sugar Level **Before**	Medication/ Insulin Dose	Blood Sugar Level **2 Hrs. After**	Physical Activity	Comments: Medication/Insulin taken How do you feel?
SUNDAY					☐ Yes ☐ No	
MEAL	Time:					
☐ Breakfast						
☐ Lunch						
☐ Dinner						
☐ Snack						

Weekly Diabetes Blood Sugar Record

Target A1C: ______ My Current A1C: ______ Target Blood Sugar Before Meals: _____

Target Blood Sugar After Meals: _____ Physical Activity Goal: ____________________

Week of: ______________		Blood Sugar Level **Before**	Medication/ Insulin Dose	Blood Sugar Level **2 Hrs. After**	Physical Activity	Comments: Medication/Insulin taken How do you feel?
MONDAY					☐ Yes ☐ No	
MEAL	Time:					
☐ Breakfast						
☐ Lunch						
☐ Dinner						
☐ Snack						
		Blood Sugar Level **Before**	Medication/ Insulin Dose	Blood Sugar Level **2 Hrs. After**	Physical Activity	Comments: Medication/Insulin taken How do you feel?
TUESDAY					☐ Yes ☐ No	
MEAL	Time:					
☐ Breakfast						
☐ Lunch						
☐ Dinner						
☐ Snack						
		Blood Sugar Level **Before**	Medication/ Insulin Dose	Blood Sugar Level **2 Hrs. After**	Physical Activity	Comments: Medication/Insulin taken How do you feel?
WEDNESDAY					☐ Yes ☐ No	
MEAL	Time:					
☐ Breakfast						
☐ Lunch						
☐ Dinner						
☐ Snack						

		Blood Sugar Level **Before**	Medication/ Insulin Dose	Blood Sugar Level **2 Hrs. After**	Physical Activity	Comments: Medication/Insulin taken How do you feel?
THURSDAY					☐ Yes ☐ No	
MEAL	Time:					
☐ Breakfast						
☐ Lunch						
☐ Dinner						
☐ Snack						
		Blood Sugar Level **Before**	Medication/ Insulin Dose	Blood Sugar Level **2 Hrs. After**	Physical Activity	Comments: Medication/Insulin taken How do you feel?
FRIDAY					☐ Yes ☐ No	
MEAL	Time:					
☐ Breakfast						
☐ Lunch						
☐ Dinner						
☐ Snack						
		Blood Sugar Level **Before**	Medication/ Insulin Dose	Blood Sugar Level **2 Hrs. After**	Physical Activity	Comments: Medication/Insulin taken How do you feel?
SATURDAY					☐ Yes ☐ No	
MEAL	Time:					
☐ Breakfast						
☐ Lunch						
☐ Dinner						
☐ Snack						
		Blood Sugar Level **Before**	Medication/ Insulin Dose	Blood Sugar Level **2 Hrs. After**	Physical Activity	Comments: Medication/Insulin taken How do you feel?
SUNDAY					☐ Yes ☐ No	
MEAL	Time:					
☐ Breakfast						
☐ Lunch						
☐ Dinner						
☐ Snack						

Weekly Diabetes Blood Sugar Record

Target A1C: ______ My Current A1C: ______ Target Blood Sugar Before Meals: ______

Target Blood Sugar After Meals: _____ Physical Activity Goal: ____________________

Week of: ______________		Blood Sugar Level **Before**	Medication/ Insulin Dose	Blood Sugar Level **2 Hrs. After**	Physical Activity	Comments: Medication/Insulin taken How do you feel?
MONDAY					☐ Yes ☐ No	
MEAL	Time:					
☐ Breakfast						
☐ Lunch						
☐ Dinner						
☐ Snack						
		Blood Sugar Level **Before**	Medication/ Insulin Dose	Blood Sugar Level **2 Hrs. After**	Physical Activity	Comments: Medication/Insulin taken How do you feel?
TUESDAY					☐ Yes ☐ No	
MEAL	Time:					
☐ Breakfast						
☐ Lunch						
☐ Dinner						
☐ Snack						
		Blood Sugar Level **Before**	Medication/ Insulin Dose	Blood Sugar Level **2 Hrs. After**	Physical Activity	Comments: Medication/Insulin taken How do you feel?
WEDNESDAY					☐ Yes ☐ No	
MEAL	Time:					
☐ Breakfast						
☐ Lunch						
☐ Dinner						
☐ Snack						

	Blood Sugar Level **Before**	Medication/ Insulin Dose	Blood Sugar Level **2 Hrs. After**	Physical Activity	Comments: Medication/Insulin taken How do you feel?
THURSDAY				☐ Yes ☐ No	
MEAL Time:					
☐ Breakfast					
☐ Lunch					
☐ Dinner					
☐ Snack					

	Blood Sugar Level **Before**	Medication/ Insulin Dose	Blood Sugar Level **2 Hrs. After**	Physical Activity	Comments: Medication/Insulin taken How do you feel?
FRIDAY				☐ Yes ☐ No	
MEAL Time:					
☐ Breakfast					
☐ Lunch					
☐ Dinner					
☐ Snack					

	Blood Sugar Level **Before**	Medication/ Insulin Dose	Blood Sugar Level **2 Hrs. After**	Physical Activity	Comments: Medication/Insulin taken How do you feel?
SATURDAY				☐ Yes ☐ No	
MEAL Time:					
☐ Breakfast					
☐ Lunch					
☐ Dinner					
☐ Snack					

	Blood Sugar Level **Before**	Medication/ Insulin Dose	Blood Sugar Level **2 Hrs. After**	Physical Activity	Comments: Medication/Insulin taken How do you feel?
SUNDAY				☐ Yes ☐ No	
MEAL Time:					
☐ Breakfast					
☐ Lunch					
☐ Dinner					
☐ Snack					

Weekly Diabetes Blood Sugar Record

Target A1C: ______ My Current A1C: ______ Target Blood Sugar Before Meals: _____

Target Blood Sugar After Meals: _____ Physical Activity Goal: ___________________

Week of: ______________		Blood Sugar Level **Before**	Medication/ Insulin Dose	Blood Sugar Level **2 Hrs. After**	Physical Activity	Comments: Medication/Insulin taken How do you feel?
MONDAY					☐ Yes	
MEAL	Time:				☐ No	
☐ Breakfast						
☐ Lunch						
☐ Dinner						
☐ Snack						
		Blood Sugar Level **Before**	Medication/ Insulin Dose	Blood Sugar Level **2 Hrs. After**	Physical Activity	Comments: Medication/Insulin taken How do you feel?
TUESDAY					☐ Yes	
MEAL	Time:				☐ No	
☐ Breakfast						
☐ Lunch						
☐ Dinner						
☐ Snack						
		Blood Sugar Level **Before**	Medication/ Insulin Dose	Blood Sugar Level **2 Hrs. After**	Physical Activity	Comments: Medication/Insulin taken How do you feel?
WEDNESDAY					☐ Yes	
MEAL	Time:				☐ No	
☐ Breakfast						
☐ Lunch						
☐ Dinner						
☐ Snack						

		Blood Sugar Level **Before**	Medication/ Insulin Dose	Blood Sugar Level **2 Hrs. After**	Physical Activity	Comments: Medication/Insulin taken How do you feel?
THURSDAY					☐ Yes ☐ No	
MEAL	Time:					
☐ Breakfast						
☐ Lunch						
☐ Dinner						
☐ Snack						
		Blood Sugar Level **Before**	Medication/ Insulin Dose	Blood Sugar Level **2 Hrs. After**	Physical Activity	Comments: Medication/Insulin taken How do you feel?
FRIDAY					☐ Yes ☐ No	
MEAL	Time:					
☐ Breakfast						
☐ Lunch						
☐ Dinner						
☐ Snack						
		Blood Sugar Level **Before**	Medication/ Insulin Dose	Blood Sugar Level **2 Hrs. After**	Physical Activity	Comments: Medication/Insulin taken How do you feel?
SATURDAY					☐ Yes ☐ No	
MEAL	Time:					
☐ Breakfast						
☐ Lunch						
☐ Dinner						
☐ Snack						
		Blood Sugar Level **Before**	Medication/ Insulin Dose	Blood Sugar Level **2 Hrs. After**	Physical Activity	Comments: Medication/Insulin taken How do you feel?
SUNDAY					☐ Yes ☐ No	
MEAL	Time:					
☐ Breakfast						
☐ Lunch						
☐ Dinner						
☐ Snack						

Weekly Diabetes Blood Sugar Record

Target A1C: ______ My Current A1C: ______ Target Blood Sugar Before Meals: ______

Target Blood Sugar After Meals: _____ Physical Activity Goal: ____________________

Week of: ______________		Blood Sugar Level **Before**	Medication/ Insulin Dose	Blood Sugar Level **2 Hrs. After**	Physical Activity	Comments: Medication/Insulin taken How do you feel?
MONDAY					☐ Yes ☐ No	
MEAL	Time:					
☐ Breakfast						
☐ Lunch						
☐ Dinner						
☐ Snack						
		Blood Sugar Level **Before**	Medication/ Insulin Dose	Blood Sugar Level **2 Hrs. After**	Physical Activity	Comments: Medication/Insulin taken How do you feel?
TUESDAY					☐ Yes ☐ No	
MEAL	Time:					
☐ Breakfast						
☐ Lunch						
☐ Dinner						
☐ Snack						
		Blood Sugar Level **Before**	Medication/ Insulin Dose	Blood Sugar Level **2 Hrs. After**	Physical Activity	Comments: Medication/Insulin taken How do you feel?
WEDNESDAY					☐ Yes ☐ No	
MEAL	Time:					
☐ Breakfast						
☐ Lunch						
☐ Dinner						
☐ Snack						

	Blood Sugar Level **Before**	Medication/ Insulin Dose	Blood Sugar Level **2 Hrs. After**	Physical Activity	Comments: Medication/Insulin taken How do you feel?
THURSDAY				☐ Yes ☐ No	
MEAL Time:					
☐ Breakfast					
☐ Lunch					
☐ Dinner					
☐ Snack					
	Blood Sugar Level **Before**	Medication/ Insulin Dose	Blood Sugar Level **2 Hrs. After**	Physical Activity	Comments: Medication/Insulin taken How do you feel?
FRIDAY				☐ Yes ☐ No	
MEAL Time:					
☐ Breakfast					
☐ Lunch					
☐ Dinner					
☐ Snack					
	Blood Sugar Level **Before**	Medication/ Insulin Dose	Blood Sugar Level **2 Hrs. After**	Physical Activity	Comments: Medication/Insulin taken How do you feel?
SATURDAY				☐ Yes ☐ No	
MEAL Time:					
☐ Breakfast					
☐ Lunch					
☐ Dinner					
☐ Snack					
	Blood Sugar Level **Before**	Medication/ Insulin Dose	Blood Sugar Level **2 Hrs. After**	Physical Activity	Comments: Medication/Insulin taken How do you feel?
SUNDAY				☐ Yes ☐ No	
MEAL Time:					
☐ Breakfast					
☐ Lunch					
☐ Dinner					
☐ Snack					

Weekly Diabetes Blood Sugar Record

Target A1C: ______ My Current A1C: ______ Target Blood Sugar Before Meals: ______

Target Blood Sugar After Meals: _____ Physical Activity Goal: ____________________

Week of: ______________		Blood Sugar Level **Before**	Medication/ Insulin Dose	Blood Sugar Level **2 Hrs. After**	Physical Activity	Comments: Medication/Insulin taken How do you feel?
MONDAY					☐ Yes ☐ No	
MEAL	Time:					
☐ Breakfast						
☐ Lunch						
☐ Dinner						
☐ Snack						
		Blood Sugar Level **Before**	Medication/ Insulin Dose	Blood Sugar Level **2 Hrs. After**	Physical Activity	Comments: Medication/Insulin taken How do you feel?
TUESDAY					☐ Yes ☐ No	
MEAL	Time:					
☐ Breakfast						
☐ Lunch						
☐ Dinner						
☐ Snack						
		Blood Sugar Level **Before**	Medication/ Insulin Dose	Blood Sugar Level **2 Hrs. After**	Physical Activity	Comments: Medication/Insulin taken How do you feel?
WEDNESDAY					☐ Yes ☐ No	
MEAL	Time:					
☐ Breakfast						
☐ Lunch						
☐ Dinner						
☐ Snack						

		Blood Sugar Level **Before**	Medication/ Insulin Dose	Blood Sugar Level **2 Hrs. After**	Physical Activity	Comments: Medication/Insulin taken How do you feel?
THURSDAY					☐ Yes ☐ No	
MEAL	Time:					
☐ Breakfast						
☐ Lunch						
☐ Dinner						
☐ Snack						
		Blood Sugar Level **Before**	Medication/ Insulin Dose	Blood Sugar Level **2 Hrs. After**	Physical Activity	Comments: Medication/Insulin taken How do you feel?
FRIDAY					☐ Yes ☐ No	
MEAL	Time:					
☐ Breakfast						
☐ Lunch						
☐ Dinner						
☐ Snack						
		Blood Sugar Level **Before**	Medication/ Insulin Dose	Blood Sugar Level **2 Hrs. After**	Physical Activity	Comments: Medication/Insulin taken How do you feel?
SATURDAY					☐ Yes ☐ No	
MEAL	Time:					
☐ Breakfast						
☐ Lunch						
☐ Dinner						
☐ Snack						
		Blood Sugar Level **Before**	Medication/ Insulin Dose	Blood Sugar Level **2 Hrs. After**	Physical Activity	Comments: Medication/Insulin taken How do you feel?
SUNDAY					☐ Yes ☐ No	
MEAL	Time:					
☐ Breakfast						
☐ Lunch						
☐ Dinner						
☐ Snack						

Weekly Diabetes Blood Sugar Record

Target A1C: ______ My Current A1C: ______ Target Blood Sugar Before Meals: ______

Target Blood Sugar After Meals: _____ Physical Activity Goal: ____________________

Week of: ______________		Blood Sugar Level **Before**	Medication/ Insulin Dose	Blood Sugar Level **2 Hrs. After**	Physical Activity	Comments: Medication/Insulin taken How do you feel?
MONDAY					☐ Yes ☐ No	
MEAL	Time:					
☐ Breakfast						
☐ Lunch						
☐ Dinner						
☐ Snack						
		Blood Sugar Level **Before**	Medication/ Insulin Dose	Blood Sugar Level **2 Hrs. After**	Physical Activity	Comments: Medication/Insulin taken How do you feel?
TUESDAY					☐ Yes ☐ No	
MEAL	Time:					
☐ Breakfast						
☐ Lunch						
☐ Dinner						
☐ Snack						
		Blood Sugar Level **Before**	Medication/ Insulin Dose	Blood Sugar Level **2 Hrs. After**	Physical Activity	Comments: Medication/Insulin taken How do you feel?
WEDNESDAY					☐ Yes ☐ No	
MEAL	Time:					
☐ Breakfast						
☐ Lunch						
☐ Dinner						
☐ Snack						

		Blood Sugar Level **Before**	Medication/ Insulin Dose	Blood Sugar Level **2 Hrs. After**	Physical Activity	Comments: Medication/Insulin taken How do you feel?
THURSDAY					☐ Yes ☐ No	
MEAL	Time:					
☐ Breakfast						
☐ Lunch						
☐ Dinner						
☐ Snack						
		Blood Sugar Level **Before**	Medication/ Insulin Dose	Blood Sugar Level **2 Hrs. After**	Physical Activity	Comments: Medication/Insulin taken How do you feel?
FRIDAY					☐ Yes ☐ No	
MEAL	Time:					
☐ Breakfast						
☐ Lunch						
☐ Dinner						
☐ Snack						
		Blood Sugar Level **Before**	Medication/ Insulin Dose	Blood Sugar Level **2 Hrs. After**	Physical Activity	Comments: Medication/Insulin taken How do you feel?
SATURDAY					☐ Yes ☐ No	
MEAL	Time:					
☐ Breakfast						
☐ Lunch						
☐ Dinner						
☐ Snack						
		Blood Sugar Level **Before**	Medication/ Insulin Dose	Blood Sugar Level **2 Hrs. After**	Physical Activity	Comments: Medication/Insulin taken How do you feel?
SUNDAY					☐ Yes ☐ No	
MEAL	Time:					
☐ Breakfast						
☐ Lunch						
☐ Dinner						
☐ Snack						

Weekly Diabetes Blood Sugar Record

Target A1C: ______ My Current A1C: ______ Target Blood Sugar Before Meals: ______

Target Blood Sugar After Meals: _____ Physical Activity Goal: ____________________

Week of: ______________		Blood Sugar Level **Before**	Medication/ Insulin Dose	Blood Sugar Level **2 Hrs. After**	Physical Activity	Comments: Medication/Insulin taken How do you feel?
MONDAY					☐ Yes ☐ No	
MEAL	Time:					
☐ Breakfast						
☐ Lunch						
☐ Dinner						
☐ Snack						
		Blood Sugar Level **Before**	Medication/ Insulin Dose	Blood Sugar Level **2 Hrs. After**	Physical Activity	Comments: Medication/Insulin taken How do you feel?
TUESDAY					☐ Yes ☐ No	
MEAL	Time:					
☐ Breakfast						
☐ Lunch						
☐ Dinner						
☐ Snack						
		Blood Sugar Level **Before**	Medication/ Insulin Dose	Blood Sugar Level **2 Hrs. After**	Physical Activity	Comments: Medication/Insulin taken How do you feel?
WEDNESDAY					☐ Yes ☐ No	
MEAL	Time:					
☐ Breakfast						
☐ Lunch						
☐ Dinner						
☐ Snack						

	Blood Sugar Level **Before**	Medication/ Insulin Dose	Blood Sugar Level **2 Hrs. After**	Physical Activity	Comments: Medication/Insulin taken How do you feel?
THURSDAY				☐ Yes ☐ No	
MEAL Time:					
☐ Breakfast					
☐ Lunch					
☐ Dinner					
☐ Snack					
	Blood Sugar Level **Before**	Medication/ Insulin Dose	Blood Sugar Level **2 Hrs. After**	Physical Activity	Comments: Medication/Insulin taken How do you feel?
FRIDAY				☐ Yes ☐ No	
MEAL Time:					
☐ Breakfast					
☐ Lunch					
☐ Dinner					
☐ Snack					
	Blood Sugar Level **Before**	Medication/ Insulin Dose	Blood Sugar Level **2 Hrs. After**	Physical Activity	Comments: Medication/Insulin taken How do you feel?
SATURDAY				☐ Yes ☐ No	
MEAL Time:					
☐ Breakfast					
☐ Lunch					
☐ Dinner					
☐ Snack					
	Blood Sugar Level **Before**	Medication/ Insulin Dose	Blood Sugar Level **2 Hrs. After**	Physical Activity	Comments: Medication/Insulin taken How do you feel?
SUNDAY				☐ Yes ☐ No	
MEAL Time:					
☐ Breakfast					
☐ Lunch					
☐ Dinner					
☐ Snack					

Weekly Diabetes Blood Sugar Record

Target A1C: ______ My Current A1C: ______ Target Blood Sugar Before Meals: ______

Target Blood Sugar After Meals: _____ Physical Activity Goal: ____________________

Week of: ______________		Blood Sugar Level **Before**	Medication/ Insulin Dose	Blood Sugar Level **2 Hrs. After**	Physical Activity	Comments: Medication/Insulin taken How do you feel?
MONDAY					☐ Yes ☐ No	
MEAL	Time:					
☐ Breakfast						
☐ Lunch						
☐ Dinner						
☐ Snack						
		Blood Sugar Level **Before**	Medication/ Insulin Dose	Blood Sugar Level **2 Hrs. After**	Physical Activity	Comments: Medication/Insulin taken How do you feel?
TUESDAY					☐ Yes ☐ No	
MEAL	Time:					
☐ Breakfast						
☐ Lunch						
☐ Dinner						
☐ Snack						
		Blood Sugar Level **Before**	Medication/ Insulin Dose	Blood Sugar Level **2 Hrs. After**	Physical Activity	Comments: Medication/Insulin taken How do you feel?
WEDNESDAY					☐ Yes ☐ No	
MEAL	Time:					
☐ Breakfast						
☐ Lunch						
☐ Dinner						
☐ Snack						

		Blood Sugar Level **Before**	Medication/ Insulin Dose	Blood Sugar Level **2 Hrs. After**	Physical Activity	Comments: Medication/Insulin taken How do you feel?
THURSDAY					☐ Yes ☐ No	
MEAL	Time:					
☐ Breakfast						
☐ Lunch						
☐ Dinner						
☐ Snack						
		Blood Sugar Level **Before**	Medication/ Insulin Dose	Blood Sugar Level **2 Hrs. After**	Physical Activity	Comments: Medication/Insulin taken How do you feel?
FRIDAY					☐ Yes ☐ No	
MEAL	Time:					
☐ Breakfast						
☐ Lunch						
☐ Dinner						
☐ Snack						
		Blood Sugar Level **Before**	Medication/ Insulin Dose	Blood Sugar Level **2 Hrs. After**	Physical Activity	Comments: Medication/Insulin taken How do you feel?
SATURDAY					☐ Yes ☐ No	
MEAL	Time:					
☐ Breakfast						
☐ Lunch						
☐ Dinner						
☐ Snack						
		Blood Sugar Level **Before**	Medication/ Insulin Dose	Blood Sugar Level **2 Hrs. After**	Physical Activity	Comments: Medication/Insulin taken How do you feel?
SUNDAY					☐ Yes ☐ No	
MEAL	Time:					
☐ Breakfast						
☐ Lunch						
☐ Dinner						
☐ Snack						

Weekly Diabetes Blood Sugar Record

Target A1C: ______ My Current A1C: ______ Target Blood Sugar Before Meals: ______

Target Blood Sugar After Meals: _____ Physical Activity Goal: ____________________

Week of: ______________		Blood Sugar Level **Before**	Medication/ Insulin Dose	Blood Sugar Level **2 Hrs. After**	Physical Activity	Comments: Medication/Insulin taken How do you feel?
MONDAY					☐ Yes ☐ No	
MEAL	Time:					
☐ Breakfast						
☐ Lunch						
☐ Dinner						
☐ Snack						
		Blood Sugar Level **Before**	Medication/ Insulin Dose	Blood Sugar Level **2 Hrs. After**	Physical Activity	Comments: Medication/Insulin taken How do you feel?
TUESDAY					☐ Yes ☐ No	
MEAL	Time:					
☐ Breakfast						
☐ Lunch						
☐ Dinner						
☐ Snack						
		Blood Sugar Level **Before**	Medication/ Insulin Dose	Blood Sugar Level **2 Hrs. After**	Physical Activity	Comments: Medication/Insulin taken How do you feel?
WEDNESDAY					☐ Yes ☐ No	
MEAL	Time:					
☐ Breakfast						
☐ Lunch						
☐ Dinner						
☐ Snack						

		Blood Sugar Level **Before**	Medication/ Insulin Dose	Blood Sugar Level **2 Hrs. After**	Physical Activity	Comments: Medication/Insulin taken How do you feel?
THURSDAY					☐ Yes	
MEAL	Time:				☐ No	
☐ Breakfast						
☐ Lunch						
☐ Dinner						
☐ Snack						
		Blood Sugar Level **Before**	Medication/ Insulin Dose	Blood Sugar Level **2 Hrs. After**	Physical Activity	Comments: Medication/Insulin taken How do you feel?
FRIDAY					☐ Yes	
MEAL	Time:				☐ No	
☐ Breakfast						
☐ Lunch						
☐ Dinner						
☐ Snack						
		Blood Sugar Level **Before**	Medication/ Insulin Dose	Blood Sugar Level **2 Hrs. After**	Physical Activity	Comments: Medication/Insulin taken How do you feel?
SATURDAY					☐ Yes	
MEAL	Time:				☐ No	
☐ Breakfast						
☐ Lunch						
☐ Dinner						
☐ Snack						
		Blood Sugar Level **Before**	Medication/ Insulin Dose	Blood Sugar Level **2 Hrs. After**	Physical Activity	Comments: Medication/Insulin taken How do you feel?
SUNDAY					☐ Yes	
MEAL	Time:				☐ No	
☐ Breakfast						
☐ Lunch						
☐ Dinner						
☐ Snack						

Weekly Diabetes Blood Sugar Record

Target A1C: _______ My Current A1C: _______ Target Blood Sugar Before Meals: ______

Target Blood Sugar After Meals: _____ Physical Activity Goal: ____________________

Week of: ________________		Blood Sugar Level **Before**	Medication/ Insulin Dose	Blood Sugar Level **2 Hrs. After**	Physical Activity	Comments: Medication/Insulin taken How do you feel?
MONDAY					☐ Yes ☐ No	
MEAL	Time:					
☐ Breakfast						
☐ Lunch						
☐ Dinner						
☐ Snack						
		Blood Sugar Level **Before**	Medication/ Insulin Dose	Blood Sugar Level **2 Hrs. After**	Physical Activity	Comments: Medication/Insulin taken How do you feel?
TUESDAY					☐ Yes ☐ No	
MEAL	Time:					
☐ Breakfast						
☐ Lunch						
☐ Dinner						
☐ Snack						
		Blood Sugar Level **Before**	Medication/ Insulin Dose	Blood Sugar Level **2 Hrs. After**	Physical Activity	Comments: Medication/Insulin taken How do you feel?
WEDNESDAY					☐ Yes ☐ No	
MEAL	Time:					
☐ Breakfast						
☐ Lunch						
☐ Dinner						
☐ Snack						

	Blood Sugar Level **Before**	Medication/ Insulin Dose	Blood Sugar Level **2 Hrs. After**	Physical Activity	Comments: Medication/Insulin taken How do you feel?
THURSDAY				☐ Yes ☐ No	
MEAL Time:					
☐ Breakfast					
☐ Lunch					
☐ Dinner					
☐ Snack					

	Blood Sugar Level **Before**	Medication/ Insulin Dose	Blood Sugar Level **2 Hrs. After**	Physical Activity	Comments: Medication/Insulin taken How do you feel?
FRIDAY				☐ Yes ☐ No	
MEAL Time:					
☐ Breakfast					
☐ Lunch					
☐ Dinner					
☐ Snack					

	Blood Sugar Level **Before**	Medication/ Insulin Dose	Blood Sugar Level **2 Hrs. After**	Physical Activity	Comments: Medication/Insulin taken How do you feel?
SATURDAY				☐ Yes ☐ No	
MEAL Time:					
☐ Breakfast					
☐ Lunch					
☐ Dinner					
☐ Snack					

	Blood Sugar Level **Before**	Medication/ Insulin Dose	Blood Sugar Level **2 Hrs. After**	Physical Activity	Comments: Medication/Insulin taken How do you feel?
SUNDAY				☐ Yes ☐ No	
MEAL Time:					
☐ Breakfast					
☐ Lunch					
☐ Dinner					
☐ Snack					

Weekly Diabetes Blood Sugar Record

Target A1C: ______ My Current A1C: ______ Target Blood Sugar Before Meals: ______

Target Blood Sugar After Meals: _____ Physical Activity Goal: ____________________

Week of: ______________		Blood Sugar Level **Before**	Medication/ Insulin Dose	Blood Sugar Level **2 Hrs. After**	Physical Activity	Comments: Medication/Insulin taken How do you feel?
MONDAY					☐ Yes ☐ No	
MEAL	Time:					
☐ Breakfast						
☐ Lunch						
☐ Dinner						
☐ Snack						
		Blood Sugar Level **Before**	Medication/ Insulin Dose	Blood Sugar Level **2 Hrs. After**	Physical Activity	Comments: Medication/Insulin taken How do you feel?
TUESDAY					☐ Yes ☐ No	
MEAL	Time:					
☐ Breakfast						
☐ Lunch						
☐ Dinner						
☐ Snack						
		Blood Sugar Level **Before**	Medication/ Insulin Dose	Blood Sugar Level **2 Hrs. After**	Physical Activity	Comments: Medication/Insulin taken How do you feel?
WEDNESDAY					☐ Yes ☐ No	
MEAL	Time:					
☐ Breakfast						
☐ Lunch						
☐ Dinner						
☐ Snack						

	Blood Sugar Level **Before**	Medication/ Insulin Dose	Blood Sugar Level **2 Hrs. After**	Physical Activity	Comments: Medication/Insulin taken How do you feel?
THURSDAY				☐ Yes ☐ No	
MEAL Time:					
☐ Breakfast					
☐ Lunch					
☐ Dinner					
☐ Snack					
	Blood Sugar Level **Before**	Medication/ Insulin Dose	Blood Sugar Level **2 Hrs. After**	Physical Activity	Comments: Medication/Insulin taken How do you feel?
FRIDAY				☐ Yes ☐ No	
MEAL Time:					
☐ Breakfast					
☐ Lunch					
☐ Dinner					
☐ Snack					
	Blood Sugar Level **Before**	Medication/ Insulin Dose	Blood Sugar Level **2 Hrs. After**	Physical Activity	Comments: Medication/Insulin taken How do you feel?
SATURDAY				☐ Yes ☐ No	
MEAL Time:					
☐ Breakfast					
☐ Lunch					
☐ Dinner					
☐ Snack					
	Blood Sugar Level **Before**	Medication/ Insulin Dose	Blood Sugar Level **2 Hrs. After**	Physical Activity	Comments: Medication/Insulin taken How do you feel?
SUNDAY				☐ Yes ☐ No	
MEAL Time:					
☐ Breakfast					
☐ Lunch					
☐ Dinner					
☐ Snack					

Weekly Diabetes Blood Sugar Record

Target A1C: ______ My Current A1C: ______ Target Blood Sugar Before Meals: _____

Target Blood Sugar After Meals: _____ Physical Activity Goal: ____________________

Week of: ______________		Blood Sugar Level **Before**	Medication/ Insulin Dose	Blood Sugar Level **2 Hrs. After**	Physical Activity	Comments: Medication/Insulin taken How do you feel?
MONDAY					☐ Yes ☐ No	
MEAL	Time:					
☐ Breakfast						
☐ Lunch						
☐ Dinner						
☐ Snack						
		Blood Sugar Level **Before**	Medication/ Insulin Dose	Blood Sugar Level **2 Hrs. After**	Physical Activity	Comments: Medication/Insulin taken How do you feel?
TUESDAY					☐ Yes ☐ No	
MEAL	Time:					
☐ Breakfast						
☐ Lunch						
☐ Dinner						
☐ Snack						
		Blood Sugar Level **Before**	Medication/ Insulin Dose	Blood Sugar Level **2 Hrs. After**	Physical Activity	Comments: Medication/Insulin taken How do you feel?
WEDNESDAY					☐ Yes ☐ No	
MEAL	Time:					
☐ Breakfast						
☐ Lunch						
☐ Dinner						
☐ Snack						

		Blood Sugar Level **Before**	Medication/ Insulin Dose	Blood Sugar Level **2 Hrs. After**	Physical Activity	Comments: Medication/Insulin taken How do you feel?
THURSDAY					☐ Yes ☐ No	
MEAL	Time:					
☐ Breakfast						
☐ Lunch						
☐ Dinner						
☐ Snack						
		Blood Sugar Level **Before**	Medication/ Insulin Dose	Blood Sugar Level **2 Hrs. After**	Physical Activity	Comments: Medication/Insulin taken How do you feel?
FRIDAY					☐ Yes ☐ No	
MEAL	Time:					
☐ Breakfast						
☐ Lunch						
☐ Dinner						
☐ Snack						
		Blood Sugar Level **Before**	Medication/ Insulin Dose	Blood Sugar Level **2 Hrs. After**	Physical Activity	Comments: Medication/Insulin taken How do you feel?
SATURDAY					☐ Yes ☐ No	
MEAL	Time:					
☐ Breakfast						
☐ Lunch						
☐ Dinner						
☐ Snack						
		Blood Sugar Level **Before**	Medication/ Insulin Dose	Blood Sugar Level **2 Hrs. After**	Physical Activity	Comments: Medication/Insulin taken How do you feel?
SUNDAY					☐ Yes ☐ No	
MEAL	Time:					
☐ Breakfast						
☐ Lunch						
☐ Dinner						
☐ Snack						

Weekly Diabetes Blood Sugar Record

Target A1C: ______ My Current A1C: ______ Target Blood Sugar Before Meals: _____

Target Blood Sugar After Meals: _____ Physical Activity Goal: ____________________

<table>
<tr><td colspan="2">Week of:
______________</td><td>Blood Sugar Level Before</td><td>Medication/ Insulin Dose</td><td>Blood Sugar Level 2 Hrs. After</td><td>Physical Activity</td><td>Comments: Medication/Insulin taken How do you feel?</td></tr>
<tr><td colspan="2">MONDAY</td><td></td><td></td><td></td><td rowspan="6">☐ Yes
☐ No</td><td rowspan="6"></td></tr>
<tr><td>MEAL</td><td>Time:</td><td></td><td></td><td></td></tr>
<tr><td>☐ Breakfast</td><td></td><td></td><td></td><td></td></tr>
<tr><td>☐ Lunch</td><td></td><td></td><td></td><td></td></tr>
<tr><td>☐ Dinner</td><td></td><td></td><td></td><td></td></tr>
<tr><td>☐ Snack</td><td></td><td></td><td></td><td></td></tr>
<tr><td colspan="2"></td><td>Blood Sugar Level Before</td><td>Medication/ Insulin Dose</td><td>Blood Sugar Level 2 Hrs. After</td><td>Physical Activity</td><td>Comments: Medication/Insulin taken How do you feel?</td></tr>
<tr><td colspan="2">TUESDAY</td><td></td><td></td><td></td><td rowspan="6">☐ Yes
☐ No</td><td rowspan="6"></td></tr>
<tr><td>MEAL</td><td>Time:</td><td></td><td></td><td></td></tr>
<tr><td>☐ Breakfast</td><td></td><td></td><td></td><td></td></tr>
<tr><td>☐ Lunch</td><td></td><td></td><td></td><td></td></tr>
<tr><td>☐ Dinner</td><td></td><td></td><td></td><td></td></tr>
<tr><td>☐ Snack</td><td></td><td></td><td></td><td></td></tr>
<tr><td colspan="2"></td><td>Blood Sugar Level Before</td><td>Medication/ Insulin Dose</td><td>Blood Sugar Level 2 Hrs. After</td><td>Physical Activity</td><td>Comments: Medication/Insulin taken How do you feel?</td></tr>
<tr><td colspan="2">WEDNESDAY</td><td></td><td></td><td></td><td rowspan="6">☐ Yes
☐ No</td><td rowspan="6"></td></tr>
<tr><td>MEAL</td><td>Time:</td><td></td><td></td><td></td></tr>
<tr><td>☐ Breakfast</td><td></td><td></td><td></td><td></td></tr>
<tr><td>☐ Lunch</td><td></td><td></td><td></td><td></td></tr>
<tr><td>☐ Dinner</td><td></td><td></td><td></td><td></td></tr>
<tr><td>☐ Snack</td><td></td><td></td><td></td><td></td></tr>
</table>

		Blood Sugar Level **Before**	Medication/ Insulin Dose	Blood Sugar Level **2 Hrs. After**	Physical Activity	Comments: Medication/Insulin taken How do you feel?
THURSDAY					☐ Yes ☐ No	
MEAL	Time:					
☐ Breakfast						
☐ Lunch						
☐ Dinner						
☐ Snack						
		Blood Sugar Level **Before**	Medication/ Insulin Dose	Blood Sugar Level **2 Hrs. After**	Physical Activity	Comments: Medication/Insulin taken How do you feel?
FRIDAY					☐ Yes ☐ No	
MEAL	Time:					
☐ Breakfast						
☐ Lunch						
☐ Dinner						
☐ Snack						
		Blood Sugar Level **Before**	Medication/ Insulin Dose	Blood Sugar Level **2 Hrs. After**	Physical Activity	Comments: Medication/Insulin taken How do you feel?
SATURDAY					☐ Yes ☐ No	
MEAL	Time:					
☐ Breakfast						
☐ Lunch						
☐ Dinner						
☐ Snack						
		Blood Sugar Level **Before**	Medication/ Insulin Dose	Blood Sugar Level **2 Hrs. After**	Physical Activity	Comments: Medication/Insulin taken How do you feel?
SUNDAY					☐ Yes ☐ No	
MEAL	Time:					
☐ Breakfast						
☐ Lunch						
☐ Dinner						
☐ Snack						

Weekly Diabetes Blood Sugar Record

Target A1C: ______ My Current A1C: ______ Target Blood Sugar Before Meals: ______

Target Blood Sugar After Meals: _____ Physical Activity Goal: ____________________

Week of: ______________	Blood Sugar Level **Before**	Medication/ Insulin Dose	Blood Sugar Level **2 Hrs. After**	Physical Activity	Comments: Medication/Insulin taken How do you feel?
MONDAY				☐ Yes ☐ No	
MEAL Time:					
☐ Breakfast					
☐ Lunch					
☐ Dinner					
☐ Snack					
	Blood Sugar Level **Before**	Medication/ Insulin Dose	Blood Sugar Level **2 Hrs. After**	Physical Activity	Comments: Medication/Insulin taken How do you feel?
TUESDAY				☐ Yes ☐ No	
MEAL Time:					
☐ Breakfast					
☐ Lunch					
☐ Dinner					
☐ Snack					
	Blood Sugar Level **Before**	Medication/ Insulin Dose	Blood Sugar Level **2 Hrs. After**	Physical Activity	Comments: Medication/Insulin taken How do you feel?
WEDNESDAY				☐ Yes ☐ No	
MEAL Time:					
☐ Breakfast					
☐ Lunch					
☐ Dinner					
☐ Snack					

		Blood Sugar Level **Before**	Medication/ Insulin Dose	Blood Sugar Level **2 Hrs. After**	Physical Activity	Comments: Medication/Insulin taken How do you feel?
THURSDAY					☐ Yes ☐ No	
MEAL	Time:					
☐ Breakfast						
☐ Lunch						
☐ Dinner						
☐ Snack						
		Blood Sugar Level **Before**	Medication/ Insulin Dose	Blood Sugar Level **2 Hrs. After**	Physical Activity	Comments: Medication/Insulin taken How do you feel?
FRIDAY					☐ Yes ☐ No	
MEAL	Time:					
☐ Breakfast						
☐ Lunch						
☐ Dinner						
☐ Snack						
		Blood Sugar Level **Before**	Medication/ Insulin Dose	Blood Sugar Level **2 Hrs. After**	Physical Activity	Comments: Medication/Insulin taken How do you feel?
SATURDAY					☐ Yes ☐ No	
MEAL	Time:					
☐ Breakfast						
☐ Lunch						
☐ Dinner						
☐ Snack						
		Blood Sugar Level **Before**	Medication/ Insulin Dose	Blood Sugar Level **2 Hrs. After**	Physical Activity	Comments: Medication/Insulin taken How do you feel?
SUNDAY					☐ Yes ☐ No	
MEAL	Time:					
☐ Breakfast						
☐ Lunch						
☐ Dinner						
☐ Snack						

Weekly Diabetes Blood Sugar Record

Target A1C: ______ My Current A1C: ______ Target Blood Sugar Before Meals: ______

Target Blood Sugar After Meals: _____ Physical Activity Goal: ____________________

Week of: ______________		Blood Sugar Level **Before**	Medication/ Insulin Dose	Blood Sugar Level **2 Hrs. After**	Physical Activity	Comments: Medication/Insulin taken How do you feel?
MONDAY					☐ Yes	
MEAL	Time:				☐ No	
☐ Breakfast						
☐ Lunch						
☐ Dinner						
☐ Snack						
		Blood Sugar Level **Before**	Medication/ Insulin Dose	Blood Sugar Level **2 Hrs. After**	Physical Activity	Comments: Medication/Insulin taken How do you feel?
TUESDAY					☐ Yes	
MEAL	Time:				☐ No	
☐ Breakfast						
☐ Lunch						
☐ Dinner						
☐ Snack						
		Blood Sugar Level **Before**	Medication/ Insulin Dose	Blood Sugar Level **2 Hrs. After**	Physical Activity	Comments: Medication/Insulin taken How do you feel?
WEDNESDAY					☐ Yes	
MEAL	Time:				☐ No	
☐ Breakfast						
☐ Lunch						
☐ Dinner						
☐ Snack						

		Blood Sugar Level **Before**	Medication/ Insulin Dose	Blood Sugar Level **2 Hrs. After**	Physical Activity	Comments: Medication/Insulin taken How do you feel?
THURSDAY					☐ Yes ☐ No	
MEAL	Time:					
☐ Breakfast						
☐ Lunch						
☐ Dinner						
☐ Snack						
		Blood Sugar Level **Before**	Medication/ Insulin Dose	Blood Sugar Level **2 Hrs. After**	Physical Activity	Comments: Medication/Insulin taken How do you feel?
FRIDAY					☐ Yes ☐ No	
MEAL	Time:					
☐ Breakfast						
☐ Lunch						
☐ Dinner						
☐ Snack						
		Blood Sugar Level **Before**	Medication/ Insulin Dose	Blood Sugar Level **2 Hrs. After**	Physical Activity	Comments: Medication/Insulin taken How do you feel?
SATURDAY					☐ Yes ☐ No	
MEAL	Time:					
☐ Breakfast						
☐ Lunch						
☐ Dinner						
☐ Snack						
		Blood Sugar Level **Before**	Medication/ Insulin Dose	Blood Sugar Level **2 Hrs. After**	Physical Activity	Comments: Medication/Insulin taken How do you feel?
SUNDAY					☐ Yes ☐ No	
MEAL	Time:					
☐ Breakfast						
☐ Lunch						
☐ Dinner						
☐ Snack						

Weekly Diabetes Blood Sugar Record

Target A1C: ______ My Current A1C: ______ Target Blood Sugar Before Meals: ______

Target Blood Sugar After Meals: _____ Physical Activity Goal: ____________________

Week of: ______________		Blood Sugar Level **Before**	Medication/ Insulin Dose	Blood Sugar Level **2 Hrs. After**	Physical Activity	Comments: Medication/Insulin taken How do you feel?
MONDAY					☐ Yes ☐ No	
MEAL	Time:					
☐ Breakfast						
☐ Lunch						
☐ Dinner						
☐ Snack						
		Blood Sugar Level **Before**	Medication/ Insulin Dose	Blood Sugar Level **2 Hrs. After**	Physical Activity	Comments: Medication/Insulin taken How do you feel?
TUESDAY					☐ Yes ☐ No	
MEAL	Time:					
☐ Breakfast						
☐ Lunch						
☐ Dinner						
☐ Snack						
		Blood Sugar Level **Before**	Medication/ Insulin Dose	Blood Sugar Level **2 Hrs. After**	Physical Activity	Comments: Medication/Insulin taken How do you feel?
WEDNESDAY					☐ Yes ☐ No	
MEAL	Time:					
☐ Breakfast						
☐ Lunch						
☐ Dinner						
☐ Snack						

		Blood Sugar Level **Before**	Medication/ Insulin Dose	Blood Sugar Level **2 Hrs. After**	Physical Activity	Comments: Medication/Insulin taken How do you feel?
THURSDAY					☐ Yes ☐ No	
MEAL	Time:					
☐ Breakfast						
☐ Lunch						
☐ Dinner						
☐ Snack						
		Blood Sugar Level **Before**	Medication/ Insulin Dose	Blood Sugar Level **2 Hrs. After**	Physical Activity	Comments: Medication/Insulin taken How do you feel?
FRIDAY					☐ Yes ☐ No	
MEAL	Time:					
☐ Breakfast						
☐ Lunch						
☐ Dinner						
☐ Snack						
		Blood Sugar Level **Before**	Medication/ Insulin Dose	Blood Sugar Level **2 Hrs. After**	Physical Activity	Comments: Medication/Insulin taken How do you feel?
SATURDAY					☐ Yes ☐ No	
MEAL	Time:					
☐ Breakfast						
☐ Lunch						
☐ Dinner						
☐ Snack						
		Blood Sugar Level **Before**	Medication/ Insulin Dose	Blood Sugar Level **2 Hrs. After**	Physical Activity	Comments: Medication/Insulin taken How do you feel?
SUNDAY					☐ Yes ☐ No	
MEAL	Time:					
☐ Breakfast						
☐ Lunch						
☐ Dinner						
☐ Snack						

Weekly Diabetes Blood Sugar Record

Target A1C: ______ My Current A1C: ______ Target Blood Sugar Before Meals: ______

Target Blood Sugar After Meals: _____ Physical Activity Goal: ____________________

Week of: ______________		Blood Sugar Level **Before**	Medication/ Insulin Dose	Blood Sugar Level **2 Hrs. After**	Physical Activity	Comments: Medication/Insulin taken How do you feel?
MONDAY					☐ Yes	
MEAL	Time:				☐ No	
☐ Breakfast						
☐ Lunch						
☐ Dinner						
☐ Snack						
		Blood Sugar Level **Before**	Medication/ Insulin Dose	Blood Sugar Level **2 Hrs. After**	Physical Activity	Comments: Medication/Insulin taken How do you feel?
TUESDAY					☐ Yes	
MEAL	Time:				☐ No	
☐ Breakfast						
☐ Lunch						
☐ Dinner						
☐ Snack						
		Blood Sugar Level **Before**	Medication/ Insulin Dose	Blood Sugar Level **2 Hrs. After**	Physical Activity	Comments: Medication/Insulin taken How do you feel?
WEDNESDAY					☐ Yes	
MEAL	Time:				☐ No	
☐ Breakfast						
☐ Lunch						
☐ Dinner						
☐ Snack						

		Blood Sugar Level **Before**	Medication/ Insulin Dose	Blood Sugar Level **2 Hrs. After**	Physical Activity	Comments: Medication/Insulin taken How do you feel?
THURSDAY					☐ Yes ☐ No	
MEAL	Time:					
☐ Breakfast						
☐ Lunch						
☐ Dinner						
☐ Snack						

		Blood Sugar Level **Before**	Medication/ Insulin Dose	Blood Sugar Level **2 Hrs. After**	Physical Activity	Comments: Medication/Insulin taken How do you feel?
FRIDAY					☐ Yes ☐ No	
MEAL	Time:					
☐ Breakfast						
☐ Lunch						
☐ Dinner						
☐ Snack						

		Blood Sugar Level **Before**	Medication/ Insulin Dose	Blood Sugar Level **2 Hrs. After**	Physical Activity	Comments: Medication/Insulin taken How do you feel?
SATURDAY					☐ Yes ☐ No	
MEAL	Time:					
☐ Breakfast						
☐ Lunch						
☐ Dinner						
☐ Snack						

		Blood Sugar Level **Before**	Medication/ Insulin Dose	Blood Sugar Level **2 Hrs. After**	Physical Activity	Comments: Medication/Insulin taken How do you feel?
SUNDAY					☐ Yes ☐ No	
MEAL	Time:					
☐ Breakfast						
☐ Lunch						
☐ Dinner						
☐ Snack						

Weekly Diabetes Blood Sugar Record

Target A1C: ______ My Current A1C: ______ Target Blood Sugar Before Meals: ______

Target Blood Sugar After Meals: _____ Physical Activity Goal: ____________________

Week of: ______________		Blood Sugar Level **Before**	Medication/ Insulin Dose	Blood Sugar Level **2 Hrs. After**	Physical Activity	Comments: Medication/Insulin taken How do you feel?
MONDAY					☐ Yes ☐ No	
MEAL	Time:					
☐ Breakfast						
☐ Lunch						
☐ Dinner						
☐ Snack						
		Blood Sugar Level **Before**	Medication/ Insulin Dose	Blood Sugar Level **2 Hrs. After**	Physical Activity	Comments: Medication/Insulin taken How do you feel?
TUESDAY					☐ Yes ☐ No	
MEAL	Time:					
☐ Breakfast						
☐ Lunch						
☐ Dinner						
☐ Snack						
		Blood Sugar Level **Before**	Medication/ Insulin Dose	Blood Sugar Level **2 Hrs. After**	Physical Activity	Comments: Medication/Insulin taken How do you feel?
WEDNESDAY					☐ Yes ☐ No	
MEAL	Time:					
☐ Breakfast						
☐ Lunch						
☐ Dinner						
☐ Snack						

	Blood Sugar Level **Before**	Medication/ Insulin Dose	Blood Sugar Level **2 Hrs. After**	Physical Activity	Comments: Medication/Insulin taken How do you feel?
THURSDAY				☐ Yes ☐ No	
MEAL Time:					
☐ Breakfast					
☐ Lunch					
☐ Dinner					
☐ Snack					

	Blood Sugar Level **Before**	Medication/ Insulin Dose	Blood Sugar Level **2 Hrs. After**	Physical Activity	Comments: Medication/Insulin taken How do you feel?
FRIDAY				☐ Yes ☐ No	
MEAL Time:					
☐ Breakfast					
☐ Lunch					
☐ Dinner					
☐ Snack					

	Blood Sugar Level **Before**	Medication/ Insulin Dose	Blood Sugar Level **2 Hrs. After**	Physical Activity	Comments: Medication/Insulin taken How do you feel?
SATURDAY				☐ Yes ☐ No	
MEAL Time:					
☐ Breakfast					
☐ Lunch					
☐ Dinner					
☐ Snack					

	Blood Sugar Level **Before**	Medication/ Insulin Dose	Blood Sugar Level **2 Hrs. After**	Physical Activity	Comments: Medication/Insulin taken How do you feel?
SUNDAY				☐ Yes ☐ No	
MEAL Time:					
☐ Breakfast					
☐ Lunch					
☐ Dinner					
☐ Snack					

Weekly Diabetes Blood Sugar Record

Target A1C: ______ My Current A1C: ______ Target Blood Sugar Before Meals: ______

Target Blood Sugar After Meals: _____ Physical Activity Goal: ____________________

Week of: ______________		Blood Sugar Level **Before**	Medication/ Insulin Dose	Blood Sugar Level **2 Hrs. After**	Physical Activity	Comments: Medication/Insulin taken How do you feel?
MONDAY					☐ Yes ☐ No	
MEAL	Time:					
☐ Breakfast						
☐ Lunch						
☐ Dinner						
☐ Snack						
		Blood Sugar Level **Before**	Medication/ Insulin Dose	Blood Sugar Level **2 Hrs. After**	Physical Activity	Comments: Medication/Insulin taken How do you feel?
TUESDAY					☐ Yes ☐ No	
MEAL	Time:					
☐ Breakfast						
☐ Lunch						
☐ Dinner						
☐ Snack						
		Blood Sugar Level **Before**	Medication/ Insulin Dose	Blood Sugar Level **2 Hrs. After**	Physical Activity	Comments: Medication/Insulin taken How do you feel?
WEDNESDAY					☐ Yes ☐ No	
MEAL	Time:					
☐ Breakfast						
☐ Lunch						
☐ Dinner						
☐ Snack						

		Blood Sugar Level **Before**	Medication/ Insulin Dose	Blood Sugar Level **2 Hrs. After**	Physical Activity	Comments: Medication/Insulin taken How do you feel?
THURSDAY					☐ Yes	
MEAL	Time:				☐ No	
☐ Breakfast						
☐ Lunch						
☐ Dinner						
☐ Snack						

		Blood Sugar Level **Before**	Medication/ Insulin Dose	Blood Sugar Level **2 Hrs. After**	Physical Activity	Comments: Medication/Insulin taken How do you feel?
FRIDAY					☐ Yes	
MEAL	Time:				☐ No	
☐ Breakfast						
☐ Lunch						
☐ Dinner						
☐ Snack						

		Blood Sugar Level **Before**	Medication/ Insulin Dose	Blood Sugar Level **2 Hrs. After**	Physical Activity	Comments: Medication/Insulin taken How do you feel?
SATURDAY					☐ Yes	
MEAL	Time:				☐ No	
☐ Breakfast						
☐ Lunch						
☐ Dinner						
☐ Snack						

		Blood Sugar Level **Before**	Medication/ Insulin Dose	Blood Sugar Level **2 Hrs. After**	Physical Activity	Comments: Medication/Insulin taken How do you feel?
SUNDAY					☐ Yes	
MEAL	Time:				☐ No	
☐ Breakfast						
☐ Lunch						
☐ Dinner						
☐ Snack						

Weekly Diabetes Blood Sugar Record

Target A1C: ______ My Current A1C: ______ Target Blood Sugar Before Meals: ______

Target Blood Sugar After Meals: _____ Physical Activity Goal: ____________________

Week of: ______________		Blood Sugar Level **Before**	Medication/ Insulin Dose	Blood Sugar Level **2 Hrs. After**	Physical Activity	Comments: Medication/Insulin taken How do you feel?
MONDAY					☐ Yes ☐ No	
MEAL	Time:					
☐ Breakfast						
☐ Lunch						
☐ Dinner						
☐ Snack						
		Blood Sugar Level **Before**	Medication/ Insulin Dose	Blood Sugar Level **2 Hrs. After**	Physical Activity	Comments: Medication/Insulin taken How do you feel?
TUESDAY					☐ Yes ☐ No	
MEAL	Time:					
☐ Breakfast						
☐ Lunch						
☐ Dinner						
☐ Snack						
		Blood Sugar Level **Before**	Medication/ Insulin Dose	Blood Sugar Level **2 Hrs. After**	Physical Activity	Comments: Medication/Insulin taken How do you feel?
WEDNESDAY					☐ Yes ☐ No	
MEAL	Time:					
☐ Breakfast						
☐ Lunch						
☐ Dinner						
☐ Snack						

		Blood Sugar Level **Before**	Medication/ Insulin Dose	Blood Sugar Level **2 Hrs. After**	Physical Activity	Comments: Medication/Insulin taken How do you feel?
THURSDAY					☐ Yes ☐ No	
MEAL	Time:					
☐ Breakfast						
☐ Lunch						
☐ Dinner						
☐ Snack						

		Blood Sugar Level **Before**	Medication/ Insulin Dose	Blood Sugar Level **2 Hrs. After**	Physical Activity	Comments: Medication/Insulin taken How do you feel?
FRIDAY					☐ Yes ☐ No	
MEAL	Time:					
☐ Breakfast						
☐ Lunch						
☐ Dinner						
☐ Snack						

		Blood Sugar Level **Before**	Medication/ Insulin Dose	Blood Sugar Level **2 Hrs. After**	Physical Activity	Comments: Medication/Insulin taken How do you feel?
SATURDAY					☐ Yes ☐ No	
MEAL	Time:					
☐ Breakfast						
☐ Lunch						
☐ Dinner						
☐ Snack						

		Blood Sugar Level **Before**	Medication/ Insulin Dose	Blood Sugar Level **2 Hrs. After**	Physical Activity	Comments: Medication/Insulin taken How do you feel?
SUNDAY					☐ Yes ☐ No	
MEAL	Time:					
☐ Breakfast						
☐ Lunch						
☐ Dinner						
☐ Snack						

Weekly Diabetes Blood Sugar Record

Target A1C: ______ My Current A1C: ______ Target Blood Sugar Before Meals: ______

Target Blood Sugar After Meals: _____ Physical Activity Goal: ____________________

Week of: ________________		Blood Sugar Level **Before**	Medication/ Insulin Dose	Blood Sugar Level **2 Hrs. After**	Physical Activity	Comments: Medication/Insulin taken How do you feel?
MONDAY					☐ Yes ☐ No	
MEAL	Time:					
☐ Breakfast						
☐ Lunch						
☐ Dinner						
☐ Snack						
		Blood Sugar Level **Before**	Medication/ Insulin Dose	Blood Sugar Level **2 Hrs. After**	Physical Activity	Comments: Medication/Insulin taken How do you feel?
TUESDAY					☐ Yes ☐ No	
MEAL	Time:					
☐ Breakfast						
☐ Lunch						
☐ Dinner						
☐ Snack						
		Blood Sugar Level **Before**	Medication/ Insulin Dose	Blood Sugar Level **2 Hrs. After**	Physical Activity	Comments: Medication/Insulin taken How do you feel?
WEDNESDAY					☐ Yes ☐ No	
MEAL	Time:					
☐ Breakfast						
☐ Lunch						
☐ Dinner						
☐ Snack						

		Blood Sugar Level **Before**	Medication/ Insulin Dose	Blood Sugar Level **2 Hrs. After**	Physical Activity	Comments: Medication/Insulin taken How do you feel?
THURSDAY					☐ Yes ☐ No	
MEAL	Time:					
☐ Breakfast						
☐ Lunch						
☐ Dinner						
☐ Snack						
		Blood Sugar Level **Before**	Medication/ Insulin Dose	Blood Sugar Level **2 Hrs. After**	Physical Activity	Comments: Medication/Insulin taken How do you feel?
FRIDAY					☐ Yes ☐ No	
MEAL	Time:					
☐ Breakfast						
☐ Lunch						
☐ Dinner						
☐ Snack						
		Blood Sugar Level **Before**	Medication/ Insulin Dose	Blood Sugar Level **2 Hrs. After**	Physical Activity	Comments: Medication/Insulin taken How do you feel?
SATURDAY					☐ Yes ☐ No	
MEAL	Time:					
☐ Breakfast						
☐ Lunch						
☐ Dinner						
☐ Snack						
		Blood Sugar Level **Before**	Medication/ Insulin Dose	Blood Sugar Level **2 Hrs. After**	Physical Activity	Comments: Medication/Insulin taken How do you feel?
SUNDAY					☐ Yes ☐ No	
MEAL	Time:					
☐ Breakfast						
☐ Lunch						
☐ Dinner						
☐ Snack						

Weekly Diabetes Blood Sugar Record

Target A1C: ______ My Current A1C: ______ Target Blood Sugar Before Meals: ______

Target Blood Sugar After Meals: _____ Physical Activity Goal: ____________________

Week of: ______________		Blood Sugar Level **Before**	Medication/ Insulin Dose	Blood Sugar Level **2 Hrs. After**	Physical Activity	Comments: Medication/Insulin taken How do you feel?
MONDAY					☐ Yes	
MEAL	Time:				☐ No	
☐ Breakfast						
☐ Lunch						
☐ Dinner						
☐ Snack						
		Blood Sugar Level **Before**	Medication/ Insulin Dose	Blood Sugar Level **2 Hrs. After**	Physical Activity	Comments: Medication/Insulin taken How do you feel?
TUESDAY					☐ Yes	
MEAL	Time:				☐ No	
☐ Breakfast						
☐ Lunch						
☐ Dinner						
☐ Snack						
		Blood Sugar Level **Before**	Medication/ Insulin Dose	Blood Sugar Level **2 Hrs. After**	Physical Activity	Comments: Medication/Insulin taken How do you feel?
WEDNESDAY					☐ Yes	
MEAL	Time:				☐ No	
☐ Breakfast						
☐ Lunch						
☐ Dinner						
☐ Snack						

	Blood Sugar Level **Before**	Medication/ Insulin Dose	Blood Sugar Level **2 Hrs. After**	Physical Activity	Comments: Medication/Insulin taken How do you feel?
THURSDAY				☐ Yes ☐ No	
MEAL Time:					
☐ Breakfast					
☐ Lunch					
☐ Dinner					
☐ Snack					

	Blood Sugar Level **Before**	Medication/ Insulin Dose	Blood Sugar Level **2 Hrs. After**	Physical Activity	Comments: Medication/Insulin taken How do you feel?
FRIDAY				☐ Yes ☐ No	
MEAL Time:					
☐ Breakfast					
☐ Lunch					
☐ Dinner					
☐ Snack					

	Blood Sugar Level **Before**	Medication/ Insulin Dose	Blood Sugar Level **2 Hrs. After**	Physical Activity	Comments: Medication/Insulin taken How do you feel?
SATURDAY				☐ Yes ☐ No	
MEAL Time:					
☐ Breakfast					
☐ Lunch					
☐ Dinner					
☐ Snack					

	Blood Sugar Level **Before**	Medication/ Insulin Dose	Blood Sugar Level **2 Hrs. After**	Physical Activity	Comments: Medication/Insulin taken How do you feel?
SUNDAY				☐ Yes ☐ No	
MEAL Time:					
☐ Breakfast					
☐ Lunch					
☐ Dinner					
☐ Snack					

Weekly Diabetes Blood Sugar Record

Target A1C: ______ My Current A1C: ______ Target Blood Sugar Before Meals: ______

Target Blood Sugar After Meals: _____ Physical Activity Goal: ____________________

Week of: ______________		Blood Sugar Level **Before**	Medication/ Insulin Dose	Blood Sugar Level **2 Hrs. After**	Physical Activity	Comments: Medication/Insulin taken How do you feel?
MONDAY					☐ Yes ☐ No	
MEAL	Time:					
☐ Breakfast						
☐ Lunch						
☐ Dinner						
☐ Snack						
		Blood Sugar Level **Before**	Medication/ Insulin Dose	Blood Sugar Level **2 Hrs. After**	Physical Activity	Comments: Medication/Insulin taken How do you feel?
TUESDAY					☐ Yes ☐ No	
MEAL	Time:					
☐ Breakfast						
☐ Lunch						
☐ Dinner						
☐ Snack						
		Blood Sugar Level **Before**	Medication/ Insulin Dose	Blood Sugar Level **2 Hrs. After**	Physical Activity	Comments: Medication/Insulin taken How do you feel?
WEDNESDAY					☐ Yes ☐ No	
MEAL	Time:					
☐ Breakfast						
☐ Lunch						
☐ Dinner						
☐ Snack						

	Blood Sugar Level **Before**	Medication/ Insulin Dose	Blood Sugar Level **2 Hrs. After**	Physical Activity	Comments: Medication/Insulin taken How do you feel?
THURSDAY				☐ Yes ☐ No	
MEAL Time:					
☐ Breakfast					
☐ Lunch					
☐ Dinner					
☐ Snack					

	Blood Sugar Level **Before**	Medication/ Insulin Dose	Blood Sugar Level **2 Hrs. After**	Physical Activity	Comments: Medication/Insulin taken How do you feel?
FRIDAY				☐ Yes ☐ No	
MEAL Time:					
☐ Breakfast					
☐ Lunch					
☐ Dinner					
☐ Snack					

	Blood Sugar Level **Before**	Medication/ Insulin Dose	Blood Sugar Level **2 Hrs. After**	Physical Activity	Comments: Medication/Insulin taken How do you feel?
SATURDAY				☐ Yes ☐ No	
MEAL Time:					
☐ Breakfast					
☐ Lunch					
☐ Dinner					
☐ Snack					

	Blood Sugar Level **Before**	Medication/ Insulin Dose	Blood Sugar Level **2 Hrs. After**	Physical Activity	Comments: Medication/Insulin taken How do you feel?
SUNDAY				☐ Yes ☐ No	
MEAL Time:					
☐ Breakfast					
☐ Lunch					
☐ Dinner					
☐ Snack					

NAME. ____

Date	AM		PM		Notes
	Blood pressure	Pulse	Blood pressure	Pulse	

BLOOD PRESSURE CATEGORY	SYSTOLIC mm Hg (upper number)	and/or	DIASTOLIC mm Hg (lower number)
NORMAL BLOOD PRESSURE	LESS THAN 120	and	LESS THAN 80
ELEVATED	120 – 129	and	LESS THAN 80
HIGH BLOOD PRESSURE (HYPERTENSION) STAGE 1	130 – 139	or	80 – 89
HIGH BLOOD PRESSURE (HYPERTENSION) STAGE 2	140 OR HIGHER	or	90 OR HIGHER
HYPERTENSIVE CRISIS (consult your doctor immediately)	HIGHER THAN 180	and/or	HIGHER THAN 120

Blood Pressure Log

Name. ____

Date	AM		PM		Notes
	Blood pressure	Pulse	Blood pressure	Pulse	

BLOOD PRESSURE CATEGORY	SYSTOLIC mm Hg (upper number)	and/or	DIASTOLIC mm Hg (lower number)
NORMAL BLOOD PRESSURE	LESS THAN 120	and	LESS THAN 80
ELEVATED	120 – 129	and	LESS THAN 80
HIGH BLOOD PRESSURE (HYPERTENSION) STAGE 1	130 – 139	or	80 – 89
HIGH BLOOD PRESSURE (HYPERTENSION) STAGE 2	140 OR HIGHER	or	90 OR HIGHER
HYPERTENSIVE CRISIS (consult your doctor immediately)	HIGHER THAN 180	and/or	HIGHER THAN 120

Blood Pressure Log

Name. ____

Date	AM		PM		Notes
	Blood pressure	Pulse	Blood pressure	Pulse	

BLOOD PRESSURE CATEGORY	SYSTOLIC mm Hg (upper number)	and/or	DIASTOLIC mm Hg (lower number)
NORMAL BLOOD PRESSURE	LESS THAN 120	and	LESS THAN 80
ELEVATED	120 – 129	and	LESS THAN 80
HIGH BLOOD PRESSURE (HYPERTENSION) STAGE 1	130 – 139	or	80 – 89
HIGH BLOOD PRESSURE (HYPERTENSION) STAGE 2	140 OR HIGHER	or	90 OR HIGHER
HYPERTENSIVE CRISIS (consult your doctor immediately)	HIGHER THAN 180	and/or	HIGHER THAN 120

Blood Pressure Log

NAME. ____

Date	AM		PM		Notes
	Blood pressure	Pulse	Blood pressure	Pulse	

BLOOD PRESSURE CATEGORY	SYSTOLIC mm Hg (upper number)	and/or	DIASTOLIC mm Hg (lower number)
NORMAL BLOOD PRESSURE	LESS THAN 120	and	LESS THAN 80
ELEVATED	120 – 129	and	LESS THAN 80
HIGH BLOOD PRESSURE (HYPERTENSION) STAGE 1	130 – 139	or	80 – 89
HIGH BLOOD PRESSURE (HYPERTENSION) STAGE 2	140 OR HIGHER	or	90 OR HIGHER
HYPERTENSIVE CRISIS (consult your doctor immediately)	HIGHER THAN 180	and/or	HIGHER THAN 120

Blood Pressure Log

Name. ____

Date	AM		PM		Notes
	Blood pressure	Pulse	Blood pressure	Pulse	

BLOOD PRESSURE CATEGORY	SYSTOLIC mm Hg (upper number)	and/or	DIASTOLIC mm Hg (lower number)
NORMAL BLOOD PRESSURE	LESS THAN 120	and	LESS THAN 80
ELEVATED	120 – 129	and	LESS THAN 80
HIGH BLOOD PRESSURE (HYPERTENSION) STAGE 1	130 – 139	or	80 – 89
HIGH BLOOD PRESSURE (HYPERTENSION) STAGE 2	140 OR HIGHER	or	90 OR HIGHER
HYPERTENSIVE CRISIS (consult your doctor immediately)	HIGHER THAN 180	and/or	HIGHER THAN 120

BLOOD PRESSURE LOG

NAME. ____

Date	AM		PM		Notes
	Blood pressure	Pulse	Blood pressure	Pulse	

BLOOD PRESSURE CATEGORY	SYSTOLIC mm Hg (upper number)	and/or	DIASTOLIC mm Hg (lower number)
NORMAL BLOOD PRESSURE	LESS THAN 120	and	LESS THAN 80
ELEVATED	120 – 129	and	LESS THAN 80
HIGH BLOOD PRESSURE (HYPERTENSION) STAGE 1	130 – 139	or	80 – 89
HIGH BLOOD PRESSURE (HYPERTENSION) STAGE 2	140 OR HIGHER	or	90 OR HIGHER
HYPERTENSIVE CRISIS (consult your doctor immediately)	HIGHER THAN 180	and/or	HIGHER THAN 120

Blood Pressure Log

Name. ____

Date	AM		PM		Notes
	Blood pressure	Pulse	Blood pressure	Pulse	

BLOOD PRESSURE CATEGORY	SYSTOLIC mm Hg (upper number)	and/or	DIASTOLIC mm Hg (lower number)
NORMAL BLOOD PRESSURE	LESS THAN 120	and	LESS THAN 80
ELEVATED	120 – 129	and	LESS THAN 80
HIGH BLOOD PRESSURE (HYPERTENSION) STAGE 1	130 – 139	or	80 – 89
HIGH BLOOD PRESSURE (HYPERTENSION) STAGE 2	140 OR HIGHER	or	90 OR HIGHER
HYPERTENSIVE CRISIS (consult your doctor immediately)	HIGHER THAN 180	and/or	HIGHER THAN 120

Blood Pressure Log

NAME. ____

Date	AM		PM		Notes
	Blood pressure	Pulse	Blood pressure	Pulse	

BLOOD PRESSURE CATEGORY	SYSTOLIC mm Hg (upper number)	and/or	DIASTOLIC mm Hg (lower number)
NORMAL BLOOD PRESSURE	LESS THAN 120	and	LESS THAN 80
ELEVATED	120 – 129	and	LESS THAN 80
HIGH BLOOD PRESSURE (HYPERTENSION) STAGE 1	130 – 139	or	80 – 89
HIGH BLOOD PRESSURE (HYPERTENSION) STAGE 2	140 OR HIGHER	or	90 OR HIGHER
HYPERTENSIVE CRISIS (consult your doctor immediately)	HIGHER THAN 180	and/or	HIGHER THAN 120

Blood Pressure Log

Name. ______________________________

Date	AM		PM		Notes
	Blood pressure	Pulse	Blood pressure	Pulse	

BLOOD PRESSURE CATEGORY	SYSTOLIC mm Hg (upper number)	and/or	DIASTOLIC mm Hg (lower number)
NORMAL BLOOD PRESSURE	LESS THAN 120	and	LESS THAN 80
ELEVATED	120 – 129	and	LESS THAN 80
HIGH BLOOD PRESSURE (HYPERTENSION) STAGE 1	130 – 139	or	80 – 89
HIGH BLOOD PRESSURE (HYPERTENSION) STAGE 2	140 OR HIGHER	or	90 OR HIGHER
HYPERTENSIVE CRISIS (consult your doctor immediately)	HIGHER THAN 180	and/or	HIGHER THAN 120

Blood Pressure Log

Name. ____

Date	AM		PM		Notes
	Blood pressure	Pulse	Blood pressure	Pulse	

BLOOD PRESSURE CATEGORY	SYSTOLIC mm Hg (upper number)	and/or	DIASTOLIC mm Hg (lower number)
NORMAL BLOOD PRESSURE	LESS THAN 120	and	LESS THAN 80
ELEVATED	120 – 129	and	LESS THAN 80
HIGH BLOOD PRESSURE (HYPERTENSION) STAGE 1	130 – 139	or	80 – 89
HIGH BLOOD PRESSURE (HYPERTENSION) STAGE 2	140 OR HIGHER	or	90 OR HIGHER
HYPERTENSIVE CRISIS (consult your doctor immediately)	HIGHER THAN 180	and/or	HIGHER THAN 120

Blood Pressure Log

Name. ____

Date	AM		PM		Notes
	Blood pressure	Pulse	Blood pressure	Pulse	

BLOOD PRESSURE CATEGORY	SYSTOLIC mm Hg (upper number)	and/or	DIASTOLIC mm Hg (lower number)
NORMAL BLOOD PRESSURE	LESS THAN 120	and	LESS THAN 80
ELEVATED	120 – 129	and	LESS THAN 80
HIGH BLOOD PRESSURE (HYPERTENSION) STAGE 1	130 – 139	or	80 – 89
HIGH BLOOD PRESSURE (HYPERTENSION) STAGE 2	140 OR HIGHER	or	90 OR HIGHER
HYPERTENSIVE CRISIS (consult your doctor immediately)	HIGHER THAN 180	and/or	HIGHER THAN 120

Blood Pressure Log

Name. ____________________

Date	AM		PM		Notes
	Blood pressure	Pulse	Blood pressure	Pulse	

BLOOD PRESSURE CATEGORY	SYSTOLIC mm Hg (upper number)	and/or	DIASTOLIC mm Hg (lower number)
NORMAL BLOOD PRESSURE	LESS THAN 120	and	LESS THAN 80
ELEVATED	120 – 129	and	LESS THAN 80
HIGH BLOOD PRESSURE (HYPERTENSION) STAGE 1	130 – 139	or	80 – 89
HIGH BLOOD PRESSURE (HYPERTENSION) STAGE 2	140 OR HIGHER	or	90 OR HIGHER
HYPERTENSIVE CRISIS (consult your doctor immediately)	HIGHER THAN 180	and/or	HIGHER THAN 120

Notes

Thank you

Thank you for your purchase!
If you enjoyed this book, please consider dropping us a review.
It takes 5 seconds and helps small businesses like ours.

Made in the USA
Monee, IL
08 November 2026

67972898R00079